Fast Fat Flush

Fasting Is the Fountain of Youth

Millan Chessman

ISBN 978-1-64559-907-4 (Paperback)
ISBN 978-1-64559-908-1 (Digital)

Covenant Books, Inc.
11661 Hwy 707
Murrells Inlet, SC 29576
www.covenantbooks.com

CONTENTS

Chapter 1:   A Reflection of My Past 7

Chapter 2:   Putting Aside Your Fear of
             Fasting 11

History of Fasting 11

Definition of a Fast 13

What is Fasting? 13

Results of Fasting 16

The What and How of a Fast 20

Twenty-four-Hour Fast 22

Kinds of Fasts 24

Juice Smoothies 29

Is Fasting Safe? 31

Intermittent Fasting 32

Ketogenic Diet 34

Preparing for a Fast 36

How to Properly Break a Fast 37
Why Fast? 39
Chapter 3:   Weight Loss and Healing 43

Percentages of Calories from Fat 45
Obesity 46
Suggestions for Weight Loss 49
Plateau 51
Scale Is Your Enemy 52

Exercise 53
Dancing Makes You Smarter 55
Chapter 4:   Cancer and Its Related Topics 58

Cancer 58
Antioxidants 61
Food 63
Benefits of a Plant-Based Diet 67
Prescription Drugs 74

Contraindications 76
Chapter 5:   Nutrients 79
Enzymes 79
Vitamins 82
Basking in Vitamin D 84
Chapter 6:   A Closer Look at Soy
Products vs. Animal Products 94

Dairy Products 94

Eating Animal Products.................... 98

Parasites.. 105

Soy Products 107

Chapter 7:   Check Out Those Ingredients... 111

Refined White Sugar 111

Food Additives 113

Chemicals 123

Salt.. 124

Exploding the Myth of the Low-Salt Diet 126

Heart Disease Deaths Four Times Higher with Low-Salt Intake 128

But Everyone Says Salt Is Bad for You… 131

Rubbing Salt into the Wound........ 131

Choose Your Salt Wisely................ 132

Wonderfully Alkaline 133

pH Alkaline Strips 133

Chapter 8:   Cleanse and Hydrate Will Exhilarate 136

What Are Colonics? 136

Colon Cleansing 138

My Suggestions for Enemas 140

Probiotics 141

Water 142

Chapter 9:   Toxic Cleanup by Fasting 148

Toxins 148

Genetically Modified or
   Genetically Engineered Foods..... 152

Organic Foods.............................. 153

Recent Diseases and the Brain 155

Chapter 10:   Spiritual Fasting....................... 164

Fasting Results.............................. 164

What Is Spiritual Fasting from
   a Biblical Perspective? 166

When Should One Fast?................. 172

Results in Fasting 172

Miracles Resulting from Those
   Who Have Fasted 173

Chapter 11:   Testimonial................... 187

CHAPTER 1

A Reflection of My Past

*No attempt should be made to cure the
body without curing the soul.*

I was a fat little girl. When I was in the seventh grade, I remember kids would call me "fatso" and "Nellie the cow." In high school, I was always thirty pounds overweight. I would go on diets, lose a few pounds, and then put the weight back on, plus more. My mother and father were both type 2 diabetics and overweight. I have a sister, two brothers, and an aunt who were all diabetics. In 1970, I was diagnosed as borderline diabetic. Looking back, I can now see that my eating was always out of control. I couldn't eat just one cookie; I had to eat the whole package. On my fifteenth birthday, my boy-friend at the time stood me up and did not come to my birthday party. I was so saddened. I ate a half gallon of ice cream all by myself. I used to eat my emotions, and it was leading me down the path to being unhealthy. Yet today, I am a senior, I am *not* a diabetic, and as healthy as can be.

I have tried practically every diet that's out there. I remember being in Overeaters Anonymous, standing in front of the group of people and saying: "Hello, my name is Millan, and I am a compulsive overeater." I thought I would be a compulsive over-eater all my life. I really believed that. At one time in my life, I was seventy pounds overweight, and I remember crying and praying, "God, *help* me."

I used to be out control with my eating habits; my cravings were all over the place. I did everything I could to stop my compulsive over-eating and weight gain. I went on Optifast, Weight Watchers, and Atkins, to name a few. I have learned that diets do not work, because they are perceived by the mind as a temporary or quick fix. I have also learned it is not *how much* I eat; it is *what* I eat and making healthy lifestyle choices.

I learned many years ago how to wean myself off of addictive sugar foods. This is what I personally did: I would place a little box of raisins in my nightstand. When the cravings came, which was around 6:00 p.m. or 7:00 p.m., I would eat the raisins. That would bring the blood glucose down. I did that every night for twenty-one days, which is the amount of time people usually need to create a habit. I finally lost the craving for sweets. I would rotate from raisins to dried mangos, dried figs, dried papaya, and prunes. If you do decide to try this, just make sure they don't have added sugar or sulfates.

After that, I would eat fresh fruit, and I had great victory over the sugar addiction. But you know what? You can also be addicted to animal products. I remember an MD who came to my health talk on fasting saying to me, "Millan, when I tried to get off eating meat, I would get weak, lethargic, and out of sorts. So I just went back to eating meat and felt so much better." I explained that it was simply his body detoxing. When you detox, you feel bad. It's called a "cleansing crisis." That is not a bad thing. Your body is dumping the poisons caused by these toxic foods, and animal products are a toxic food and very addictive. That's why one feels so out of sorts. It takes time, and one must trust the process.

People tend to be unhealthy mainly because they do not have the knowledge and application of how to be healthy. However, this is not always the case, as I know some people who simply do not want to know and instead take prescription drugs to remedy their health issues. I had not a clue as to why I was borderline diabetic in 1970. When I did my first fast and cleanse, it gave me an awareness of the abuse that I was doing to my body without even realizing it, thinking that eating the standard American diet was adequate for my health needs. When I changed my diet and started fasting on a regular basis, I had complete control over my appetite, my way of thinking, my ambitions, and my health. I never realized the importance of eating God-made natural foods. Knowledge really is power.

CHAPTER 2

Putting Aside Your Fear of Fasting

Fasting regularly will result in joy and gladness.

—Zechariah 8:19

History of Fasting

The concept of fasting is not a new one; however, it has been ignored in our society for quite some time. Hippocrates, our first doctor, recommended fasting to recover from sickness, and I believe being overweight is definitely a sickness. "Everyone has a doctor in him," said Hippocrates, who lived four hundred years before Christ. He, as well as Galen and all the other physicians of ancient times, advocated fasting. Others such as Plato and Socrates felt they always obtained mental efficiency through fasting. Fasting has been man's oldest and best method of improving health for thousands of years. In ancient times, fasting was administered when one became ill. When I traveled in Greece, we visited ancient fasting communities where those that were ill stayed and only drank water until they recuperated and felt wonderful and full of energy. Isn't it amazing that when one fasts, the body immediately starts to heal? I have seen this numerous times in cases of cancer, diabetes, and high blood pressure; the list is numerous. See my testimonials.

Fasting is the quickest way to regain optimum health; it impressively raises the white blood cell count, which stimulates stem-cell-based regeneration in renewal of immune system cells. In a preliminary study, it was discovered that cancer patients who fasted for seventy-two hours before chemotherapy were protected from the toxic results of the treatment.

Definition of a Fast

I looked up the word "fast" in *Webster's* dictionary, and it read, "To abstain from all foods." Please know that fasting is *not starvation*. On my fasting programs, you will not starve to death. A very important aspect of fasting is the amount of water you drink. (See my water topic in chapter 8.)

What is Fasting?

Fasting is not a diet, and fasting is not a fad. Fasting is only one component to the whole program of a healthy lifestyle; however, it is a very important one. Fasting gives control over the flesh and clears the mind. Now, my brain tells my body what to do. In other words, I have control. That's what fasting does. It gives you control, ultimately leading to good health.

Fasting is the ability to cleanse the palate, change your eating patterns, detox the body, promote self-healing, and, most importantly, lose weight. Fasting is one of the most effective natural methods of rebuilding the body's own dynamic healing powers and overcoming many major ailments. Studies show that a fast can change stem cells from seclusion to activation. Doctors will recommend it for patients afflicted with colds and many diseases. You will find that when you go without food, the body kicks in to rid itself of the sickness and fat. I tell you as passionately as I know how: incorporate a regular fasting program in your life, and you will never forget me because it will change your life! You will finally have control over your beautiful body. For once in your life, your mind tells your body, "I am in control. You will do as I tell you." That is great victory! If you fast on a regular basis, so much change will happen in your life. Besides the weight coming off, you will have a different attitude, a different outlook, and a closer walk with the Creator of the universe, feel better, look better, and will build a stronger immune system, which means less sickness and disease. You will even look younger!

More and more research shows that sporadic fasting could have lasting benefits. "Fasting alone is more powerful in preventing and reversing some diseases than drugs," says Satchidananda Panda, an associate professor of regulatory biology at the Salk Institute for Biological Studies in San Diego, California.

Scientists recently revealed that people on "feast-and-famine" diets could live longer lives. Ancient hunter-gatherers often ate only sporadically, the researchers noted in their article. This suggests that the ability to function at a high level both physically and mentally during extended periods without food may have been crucial in human evolution and that the human body may have adapted to perform at its best with sporadic fasting. Such sporadic fasting could consist of eating five hundred calories or less either two days each week, or every other day, or not eating breakfast and lunch several days each week, the researchers said.

I have an interest in history and the World War II Holocaust and have read about the starvation in the death camps. These people were so hungry they would steal, kill, and sell their bodies, decisions they would not normally make, to get a slice of bread. I tell my clients this: I believe when we have another famine, and we will, just look at history, those of us who fast on a regular basis will be the survivors. We will be able to share the little food we get with others. Why? Because we will have control over our flesh and have control over the desire to eat. Our bodies will be so used to going without food regularly, simply because we are creatures of habit and our body does what we train it to do if we do it regularly. These times of famine will not affect us as they would others.

Prior research suggests that in animals, sporadic fasting can fend off or even reverse such illnesses as cancer, diabetes, heart disease, and neurodegenerative disorders. Animal studies suggest that sporadic fasting provides these benefits by allowing the body to respond better to stress that might otherwise damage it. For example, fasting could shrink tumors, reduce inflammation, or improve the removal of damaged molecules and other components of cells, the researchers said. "Sporadic fasting helps the body to rejuvenate and repair, thereby promoting overall health," Panda told *Live Science.* Because of this, you can expect to have better health for the rest of your life.

Results of Fasting

I did my first fast when I was twenty-nine years old. I took cleansing herbs, did enemas, and drank juices. I was shocked when I saw these, what I call, "poopoo monsters" come out of my body. I thought,

My gosh, if I have this inside me, others must as well. At that time, I searched everywhere for books on cleansing and fasting but found only two. One was *Become Younger*, by Dr. Norman Walker, who lived to be 118 years old according to his family members. The other book was *Bowel Management and Tissue Cleansing*, by Dr. Bernard Jensen. Later, I did another fast which resulted in a backache so bad that I could not straighten my back and I could hardly walk. Even the chiropractor was unable to help me. At the time, I was confused, but now I know it was simply a cleansing crisis. I did another seven-day fast, and this time, I had backache, but not as intense. Now, when I fast, I don't have any backaches, only light headaches and lethargy.

Expect to have bad breath initially, as well as dark yellow urine, and your pH test to read acidic. Those who have used a lot of hallucinogenic drugs can anticipate a duplication of their effects as the stored drugs reenter the bloodstream. Since your skin is the largest eliminator of toxins and poisons, you may have some pimples, rashes, even boils as you go through the process. This is a normal cleansing aspect of the fast. This is a good time to introduce yourself to a Korean body scrub.

When you start a fast, the first seventy-two hours can be a struggle because you will be hungry. I tell my clients to just go to bed. If you are a Christian, you can take authority over the hunger and command it to leave your mind "in the name of Jesus of Nazareth." That is what I do, and trust me, the hunger is *gone*! Will it come back again? It can. Just repeat the same command, and you might say The Lord's Prayer. I say: "the Lord is my shepherd, I shall not want." Pretty soon, the hunger won't come back.

During the first seventy-two hours, it is a good idea to be in an atmosphere where you can rest. Lie down with TV off. Or just go to bed! More nutrients will reach the inner cells, and waste elimination will improve. Ultimately, you will naturally eat less because more of the nutrients will be made available.

I have had clients that have done fasts and actually ended up looking ten years younger. I remember doing a twenty-one-day fast myself and found that one day, I had some lines and the next day they were gone. Hard to believe, but I tell you it is the truth!

There are so many weight loss programs that are seriously harmful to your body; one that comes to mind is the high-animal-protein weight loss diet. Please refer to chapter 6 on the effects of animal protein. Unlike these programs, fasting can benefit your mind as well as your body and soul.

Benefits of Fasting

The following was taken from Paul Bragg's book, *Miracle of Fasting*.

- Fasting rids the body of toxins, giving it an internal cleansing shower.
- Fasting does not deprive the body of essential nutrients.
- Fasting can be used to uncover the sources of food allergies.
- Fasting is used effectively in the treatment of schizophre-nia and other mental illnesses.
- Fasting under proper supervision can be tolerated easily for many weeks.
- Fasting does not accumulate appetite; hunger pangs disappear in seventy-two hours.

- Fasting is routine for most of the animal kingdom.
- Fasting has been a common practice since the beginning of man's existence.
- Fasting is a rite in all religions; the Bible alone has seventy-four references to fasting.
- Fasting under proper conditions is absolutely safe.
- Fasting is a blessing.
- Fasting is not starving; it's nature's cure that God has given us.

Millan adds:

- Fasting increases the libido.
- Fasting rids the mind of depression.
- Fasting puts cancer in remission.
- Fasting rids the body of diabetes.
- Fasting is instructed by God.
- Fasting is safe.
- Fasting can reverse the aging process.

The What and How of a Fast

Isn't it exciting to know that a juice smoothie fast will take an average of one pound a day off your body in total, amounting to fourteen-pound loss in fourteen days? Of course, you do have to take into consideration how much one weighs and their age. There is a bonus as well, and that is that the body starts a healing process and you can actually look younger!

There are so many benefits to fasting. There are many diseases that have been healed from fasting, diseases such as schizophrenia, Parkinson's, gonorrhea, syphilis, MS, cancer, and diabetes, just to name a few. I don't know of one disease that has not been remedied with a fast. Most people that have fasted stated that they had more energy, vitality, and clarity of mind, felt stronger, and looked younger after they completed their fast.

For most people, it is easier to reduce weight by fasting than by cutting down on foods, as most weight loss diets require. Fasting keeps the hunger to a minimum, except during the first seventy-two hours, while it takes inches and pounds off the body. It does this more quickly than any weight loss program. Fast at a time when you know you can rest, especially the first twenty-four to seventy-two hours. Do it on a day that you have off of work. That way, you can rest and experience the cleansing crisis. Remember, as you continue to fast you, will experience chills and little coolness, so if you can fast when the weather is a little warmer, that makes it more pleasant. Rest is very important. Do not push yourself to do any strenuous exercise. Be sure to take hot baths and scrub your skin with a loofah brush for five minutes before taking your bath. If you must read, read a book on fasting or read something positive like the Bible, especially the book of John. When you begin a fast that will continue longer than twenty-four hours, it is important to eat fruits and vegetables three days before you begin the fast.

Twenty-four-Hour Fast

Here are some tips on how to do a twenty-four-hour fast: eat your big meal at 11:00 a.m. This meal should consist of some starch, some substance like potato, sweet potato, corn, beans, quinoa, fruits and vegetables, and some nuts and seeds. Eat those foods until your tummy is full. Then make a plan. Retire early, no TV, no company, and no activities. Read a book on fasting. Drink plenty of water. If you're really hungry at five o'clock, drink 1 1/2 cups of hot vegetable broth, which will cut your appetite immediately. Go to bed early. Even if you don't sleep, go to bed. The next morning, get up. Drink something hot such as tea, coffee, or even simply hot water. The heat of that liquid will start your digestive system, and you will have a good elimination.

Continue to drink plenty of water throughout the day. If you are struggling with hunger, drink two eight-ounce glasses of water, all down at the same time. That will kill your appetite. Then just rest. Before you know it, it is eleven o'clock in the morning, and it has been twenty-four hours.

Be sure to do this faithfully once every week. I do my fast on Mondays. You do your fast when you know you can rest without disturbances. If you do this consistently, you will discover not only weight loss, but you will discover control over your flesh, your skin will look glowing, you will have a sense of well-being, and there is a certain amount of contentment knowing you have completed this fast once every week. After about a month, you can go into a three-day fast or a seven-day fast very easily. Just remember this when you are doing this fast and you are struggling with food thoughts: "this too shall pass." Sometimes, I need to say this multiple times, but it works. Or I take authority over my food thoughts, and I command them to depart from my brain in the name of Jesus.

Kinds of Fasts

There are four kinds of fasting choices I offer at my fasting retreat: fruit and vegetable juice fast, water fast, lemonade fast (also known as the Master Cleanse), and green smoothie fast. In the old days, water fasts were advocated. People ask, "Which should I do?" Here are my suggestions: If you have never fasted before, first try a vegetable or fruit juice smoothie fast. Allow yourself three ten-ounce glasses each day, one fruit, and two vegetable juices. The vegetable smoothie fast consists of carrots, beets, spinach, celery, red cabbage, cucumber, and parsley and has complete nutrition. The fruit smoothie con-sists of frozen banana, apple, blueberry, raspberry, blackberry, grapes, and cantaloupe with the juice of pineapple/coconut juice blended completely. You can do sixteen to thirty-two ounces of the vegetable juice smoothie and ten ounces of the fruit smoothie each day. If you get hungry around 5:00 p.m. or 6:00 p.m., boil one mug of distilled water and put a rounded teaspoon of organic Better Than Bouillon vegetable broth and stir completely. Those of you that like spice, place a few drops of Tabasco sauce in broth. It is very delicious! I guarantee it will cut your appetite completely.

Do a fast on the day when you can rest. That is so very important, because if you have never fasted, you may get lethargic, have headaches, and feel weak. I remember my gym instructor did a lemonade fast, and she still did step aerobics and said she had a lot of energy. This does not happen to me, though everyone is different. If you have never fasted before, please expect to feel tired and listless and have headaches. Go to bed and, please, no TV.

Dr. Otto Buchinger has supervised over 80,000 fasts, and he advocates juice fasts as opposed to water fasts; he had no knowledge of "lemonade fasts" or "green smoothie" fasts in his time. He states that people will recover more quickly from disease and more effectively in cleansing and rejuvenation of the tissues with the juice fast than they will with the water fast. I say the green smoothie fast is equivalent nutrition-wise to the juice fast.

Dick Gregory went on a liquid fast for over thirty months. He ran at least three miles daily. To celebrate the one hundredth day of the fruit juice fast, he ran fifteen miles. He informed us that he would drink one gallon of fresh juice one day and the following day one gallon of distilled water. He did about three years of purification and fruitarian diet before he achieved optimum energy on this liquid fast. He ran twenty miles in the Boston marathon race.

Those of you who have never fasted, please do not start on a water fast. It may be too radical. Do the juice smoothie first. Start slowly with the twenty-four-hour fast, and then you can work into a seven-day fast after a few weeks of doing the twenty-four-hour fast. Over time, your body will get used to not eating. I also recommend doing a cleansing herbal program with your fast. Why? Because it will make you feel full, and you will see so much ugly waste come out of your body.

A client once told me what she experienced when she went to a water-only fast retreat. She said, "I stayed for ten days, drank only water, and became very constipated. I came home and could not eliminate. You feel like something is there but won't come out. Normally I don't have this problem. After one and a half weeks, I needed to go for a colonic to get back to normal. I lost my hair when I was there." This is why I professionally suggest that while you fast, you to do colon cleansing and take cleansing herbs to avoid these negative results. Your fast will produce quicker, and better, results while you go through the process.

A water fast can seem very radical, and be difficult, for those who have been eating poorly for a while. I suggest starting your journey to health with a juice smoothie fast; you will be getting incredible nutrients, far more than you did when you were eating all the unhealthy foods that caused your poor health in the first place. It will consist of more vitamins, minerals, and enzymes than you've ever had in the past.

Now that I have done so much fasting, I do the lemonade fast. I love the taste, especially the cayenne. It will give some people more energy! However, a water fast is more intense, and you will detox more quickly. Please be sure to drink only distilled water (see chapter 8). I recommend a water fast for those that have done much fasting in the past. As always, be sure to drink two liters of water each day.

"On which program will I lose more weight?" one may ask. If you have weight to lose, you will lose weight on all of the above fasts. More than likely, you will lose more weight on the water fast, but again, don't do it if you have never done a fast.

The lemonade fast is the second best fast on which to lose more weight. The third is the veggie, fruit smoothie fast, which is both comparable as far as weight loss is concerned.

Can you fast periodically for the rest of your life? Absolutely, you can. I have been fasting for forty years off and on; it has become a part of my life. I fast every week for twenty-four hours and then fast for three to seven days once every six months. I say that passionately and enthusiastically. Fasting can be a part of your life as it has been in mine. Fasting is the fountain of youth! Remember, this is what Hippocrates advocated thousands of years ago for optimum health and to treat sickness and disease.

Years ago, I was diagnosed with a positive pap smear. I had another pap done just to make sure, and again it came back positive. I was urged by the MD to get my cervix cauterized. I refused and instead did a seven-day fast, taking cleansing herbs, colon cleansing, and juices. I then went back to the MD, did another pap smear, and it came back negative. Since then, I have seen this happen to two of my clients that made the same decision. Now that I fast regularly, it keeps my body under control and much more healthy.

Juice Smoothies

I had a client who stayed at my fasting retreat share with me the dramatic improvement he experienced doing green juice smoothies. He'd had hepatitis C since 1995. Hepatitis C is indicative of liver damage and liver cells dying. He started on the regimen of drinking green juice smoothies every day. About three months later, he had his liver enzymes tested. They were normal! Prior to drinking the green smoothies, these test results were very high. I think it is a miracle!

When my husband was alive, he had severe insomnia. Many people drinking the green smoothies have resolved their insomnia condition. Studies show those who suffer from chronic insomnia actually have brain cell damage. These are the folks that develop dementia and Alzheimer's disease later in life. Another great benefit of the green smoothies is all of the chlorophyll, which is important to rid the body of odors and keep it clean in all areas. Probably most important to those wanting to lose weight is that chlorophyll will stabilize the blood sugar level. This is so important for those with sugar cravings. You will find that you want to eat more of the God-made natural foods and less of the junk foods that are a detriment to your health. That's called victory! Another great benefit of drinking the green smoothies is the nutrient assimilation, which is so important to weight loss and future weight control.

One of the reasons people are overweight is because they are actually starving for nutrients. They feel full but are still hungry and continue eating. The juice smoothies not only resolve this problem, but they also provide the body with more oxygen, in which we are immensely deficient. We only get 20 percent of the oxygen our bodies actually need. Oxygen is important to keep parasites away and desperately needed by the brain for proper function. Your bowels will move more frequently, which increases weight loss! One person stated that she lost nine pounds within a month just from drinking smoothies and doing no other weight loss program!

My preparation of the green smoothie is as follows: I get organic spring greens, blend two large handfuls with three dates, one frozen banana, and one liter plus one cup of ice-cold distilled water in blender until completely liquefied. You can add orange juice, organic kale, organic spinach, celery, peeled cucumber, and dried fruit, such as apricots, papaya, mango, and berries. It may take some folks a while to acclimate to the taste, but hang in there, and you will love it! Why? Because you have so much more energy and lose weight, and any health issues may go away completely! No more naps in the afternoon, and your immune system is way up there with a high alkaline level. Others have stated they feel better mentally, with very little stress. Junk food cravings were gone, their appetite seemed to be in control, and their eating was especially lessened. Drink your smoothies until the day you die; it will slow the aging process. As you enjoy your smoothies, be sure to rotate your veggies.

Is Fasting Safe?

Fasting won't hurt people, provided they maintain an adequate fluid intake. However, fasting entirely for long periods of time can be harmful. Your body needs a variety of vitamins, minerals, and other nutrients from food to stay healthy. Not getting enough of these nutrients during fasting programs can lead to symptoms such as fatigue, dizziness, constipation, dehydration, gallstones, and cold intolerance. It is possible to die if you fast too long.

Women who are pregnant or breastfeeding should not fast. Before you go on any type of new diet, particularly one that involves fasting, talk to a health practitioner who knows about fasting to find out whether it is safe and appropriate for you.

Intermittent Fasting

Intermittent fasting is a very popular dieting program today. But as I have been saying in this book, diets do not work, and I consider intermittent fasting a diet and lump it into that category. Why? Because when you get off this program (diet), you risk the chance of reaping a ravenous appetite, and there you go eating out of control. This type of fasting does not give the body a complete opportunity to detox effectively in order to obtain optimum health and stop the cravings! Isn't that what you really want ultimately? Losing weight and keeping it off begin that journey if done properly. With this intermittent fasting, much discussion is made on zero carbs prior to beginning intermittent fasting. Remember, there are two different kinds of carbohydrates. There are the refined carbohydrates, and there are the complex carbs. Your body thrives and desperately needs complex carbs. Don't throw the baby out with the bath water. Your body naturally needs complex carbs to exist. Glucose will be produced which is important for your blood glucose level, ultimately obtaining the energy you so desperately need and producing optimum health.

In my fasting program, I had a client who did a seven-day fast with the decision to continue when she got home. At home, she went through a major cleansing crisis. Upon the effects of the crisis, she broke her fast without proper counsel and guidance. Those impurities are still in the body. See Paul Braggs testimonial in his book *Miracle of Fasting*. He planned to do a thirty-day fast, and on day twenty-one, he released almost pure dichlorodiphenyltrichloroethane (DDT) in his urine. Had he broke his fast on day twenty, he would not have passed the DDT.

I offer psyllium to take. This assists greatly in curbing the appetite. At the same time, the body is detoxifying. The body needs natural sugars. And I am an advocate of fresh fruit. This is what I call a god made food. It should always be a part of your diet. Yes, these diets, including the paleo, will result in weight loss, but sooner or later, you gain back the weight and *more*. Eating God-made foods, fruits, veggies, grains, legumes, and raw nuts and seeds and doing a cardio exercise will keep your weight off for the rest of your life, and as stated before it's not how much you eat, it's what you eat. I use the palm of my hand as a guide; eating a handful of raw nuts and seeds, all the veggies and legumes I want, four fruits, and I allow myself two breads daily.

Remember, after seventy-two hours of fasting, the body will lose its appetite for food. I remember my father always said anything worthwhile requires effort, focus, and determination. Cells are made afresh and new through fasting.

Ketogenic Diet

There is such hype on the need for animal protein, and many trainers and gyms recommend ingesting 230 to 250 grams of animal protein, but I recommend 25 to 35 grams of plant protein. Keep in mind that there is plenty of protein in veggies and legumes. I have not eaten animal protein since 1989. No American has ever died for lack of protein in the United States.

The ketogenic diet is another word for Atkins diet. I did the Atkins diet back in the 1970s. I lost a lot of weight. I have struggled with obesity most of my life as I stated earlier. But when I went off the Atkins diet, I not only gained all my weight back, but I gained more than before.

New research at the European Society of Cardiology Congress in Germany found that diets very low in carbs may raise individuals' risks of premature death over time. Coauthor Maciej Banach, president of the Polish Mother's Memorial Hospital Research Institute, said to *Times*. "We should avoid diets with extremely low and very low levels of carbs, specifically those that draw less than 26% of daily calorie intake from carbs. Always eat complex carbs for longevity. Cutting out carbs is simply not healthy. Data from almost 25,000 people collected through the National Health and Nutrition Examination Survey between 1999 and 2010 found that over an average of 6.4 years of follow-up people who consumed the lowest amount of carbs had a 32 percent higher risk of total mortality, a roughly 50 percent higher risk of dying from vascular diseases and a higher risk of dying from cancer, compared to people who ate the most carbs." I truly believe this is because we are not created to eat animals. We have the digestive system of the herbivore twenty to twenty-two feet of small intestine and five to five and a half feet of large intestine. That is why I have seen so many colons impacted with waste that has built up over the years of eating fish, chicken, beef, pork eggs, and dairy. These products have *no* fiber!

Preparing for a Fast

Three days prior to starting your fast, eat only fruits and vegetables. Aim to drink at least two liters of water each day and be sure not to be around where there is the aroma of food or food itself. Don't tell anyone that you are going to partake in a fast. If you tell others, such as family and friends, that you are fasting or going to go on a fast, you may get much ridicule, criticism, or argument about your choice. They may not understand this subject and may think you are going to starve to death and, in the process, do great damage to your body. Of course, that is not true. Talk with a health practitioner who knows about fasting and its benefits and let him be your guide if you desire. If you discuss this with a doctor, be sure this doctor is knowledgeable in the area of fasting. If he is not, trust me, he *will* discourage you from fasting. Otherwise, consider keeping it to yourself.

How to Properly Break a Fast

On the third or fourth day after breaking a fast, you can become ravenous. Be very careful and sensitive to your appetite. The first couple of days aren't bad, but around the third day, *bam,* it can hit you. I tell my clients to make a plan. One thing you know when you get up in the morning: you will be eating. Do you have healthy foods in your refrigerator? Where will you be around 5:00 p.m.? Put some raw nuts or seeds or a health bar in the glove compartment of your car, so that if you happen to be driving around and the hunger hits, you will be prepared, and you won't pull into a fast food joint and order French fries. Always be prepared, and, again, I repeat: plan your day for what you are going to eat. If you fasted six days or longer, break your fast on raw fruits and veggies for four days. Then you can add cooked foods. This will help in controlling a massive hunger attack you could experience.

I have always felt that eating breakfast was not a healthy decision; however, we have been told in our society that it is important to start your day with a good breakfast. My breakfast consists of one quart of green juice smoothie, consisting of vegetables and fruit. I eat only twice a day, and I end my day eating fruit or dried fruit.

Remember, your stomach is about the size of a fist, or it should be. Everything you eat, except raw veggies or salad, should be able to fit into the palm of your hand as a general rule. Normally, I state, "It is not how much you eat, it is what you eat," such as "God-made foods"; fruits, vegetables, grains, legumes, and raw nuts and seeds. When you break a fast, you certainly don't want to gorge yourself. So if you do a twenty-four-hour fast, you can break it eating these God-made natural foods. If you break a seven-day fast, you want to eat fruits on days eight and nine, add vegetables on days nine and ten, then on day eleven, and so on, you can add the grains, legumes, and raw nuts and seeds. If you do a fourteen-day fast, then on days fifteen and sixteen eat only fruits, on days seventeen and eighteen add vegetables, and on day nineteen and so on, you can add the grains, legumes, and raw nuts and seeds. To keep healthy and disease-free for the rest of your life, only eat these foods, in juice form or otherwise, and nothing else. This is the perfect diet. When you break a fast with the exception of a twenty-four-hour fast for four days after, eat your fruit and veggies raw. If you start by eating cooked food, you will find yourself ravenous around the third day. You don't want that to happen.

Why Fast?

Without your health, you have nothing. You can't work, and you can't be loving to your family, spouse, and friends. Riches, fame, and possessions are completely meaningless without your health. It is the most important possession you can have, and frankly, people really don't want to be around you or you become a burden to others, which is a shame.

What is so very sad is that people really don't know how to be healthy. I hear all the time: "Oh, I eat healthy," but when you ask in detail what they eat, these foods are not healthy. People get their information from their doctors who mostly prescribe toxic prescription drugs and diagnose health issues. Their knowledge of diet, health, and nutrition is minimal. Listen, the most important health decision you can make is what you are putting into your body. There are four steps to perfect health: diet, detox, exercise, and vitamin/mineral supplements. Fasting is in the category of "detox," because when you fast, your body starts to flush out toxins. Have you watched an older person walking? Their bodies are so full of impurities that they can hardly bend without feeling pain.

The mystery of fasting will never be understood completely, but it accomplishes an antiaging result, rejuvenation of the body, and cleansing and renewing so many different organs of the body. Here is a quote from Edward Humphrey: "True wisdom is to know what is best worth knowing and to do what is best worth doing."

When anyone abstains totally from food, incredible changes will happen. These changes revise attitudes about food and put the appetite in check with the body's real need for energy. Your body is incredible. If you can give it any boost of help, it will respond and become healthy and obesity-free. I believe those who fast on a regular basis have better mental clarity, memory retention, and self-control in all areas of their lives. After a couple of days of fasting, your body will produce ketones, which are a very important appetite suppressant.

Dr. Cott says that the rate at which you lose weight is generally in proportion to the degree to which you are overweight. Most people who fast for a week can expect to lose up to twenty pounds, but when you fast, it's not unusual to lose four to six pounds the first day and even as much as ten pounds in four days. The general rule is that overweight people lose weight at a faster rate than thin people do during a fast. Most of the weight that you lose initially is water. So during the first five days of the fast, the body will dump an excess of impurities, toxins, and fluids.

When you fast, your body is releasing all the diseased tissue. Your body will be releasing all the infected tissue and, therefore, building up your immune system. By fasting on a regular basis, you can fight off illness and the degenerative diseases that are so common in this polluted world in which we live. If you feel sickness coming on or you feel listless or depressed, go on a fast. That's the best thing you can do for your body. Each time you fast, you feel better and better because your body is healing itself and rebuilding its immune system.

People think that they need to eat regularly to keep their blood sugar constant, but a healthy body does that even when you are not eating at all. I will hear quite often people say, "I cannot fast because I have hypoglycemia," which is when blood sugar level is too low. Their body is going to go into fasting mode just like anyone else's, and they're going to experience headaches, lethargy, etc. I myself was a borderline diabetic in 1970 and have done numerous fasts with great success. So we cannot use that as an excuse not to fast. When you fast, your body is forced to dip into the energy that it stores to get what it needs to keep you going so you will lose weight. If you do a fast for weight loss purposes and you break the fast and go back to eating the foods that caused you to be overweight to begin with, you will have defeated the purpose of fasting. What you need to remember is that fasting is one component to this weight loss program. Eating a plant-based diet and God-made foods and drinking at least two liters of purified water daily are so important. This will help you to maintain your weight loss and continue to give you victory over your appetite. So I recommend periodic fasts. This gives you control over your appetite when you break the fast and transition into eating a plant-based diet.

---CHAPTER 3---

Weight Loss and Healing

Fasting is necessary for overcoming spiritual attacks.

—Mark 9:29

In this book, I want to focus on the area of weight loss using the method of fasting. When I hear people tell me they have lost three pounds in one day from fasting and internal cleansing, I am still amazed. People will ask, "How much weight or how many inches can I expect to lose?" The amount of weight a person loses from fasting really depends on their age, how toxic their bodies are, and how overweight they are. All of this will determine how much weight they will lose. For example, if a person is forty pounds overweight and they are fifty years old, doing either a seven-day fast using juices, green smoothies, Master Cleanse, or water, they can expect to lose about one pound a day. So by the end of the week, they would have lost seven to ten pounds. Remember, I am generalizing. Fasting is a very wonderful way of keeping your weight down, staying in control of your eating, being sensitive to health issues, staying healthy, and keeping your alkaline/pH level where it is supposed to be.

I also want to emphasize not to weigh yourself daily. Unfortunately, when a person gets on a scale every day, the scale can deceive them into thinking they have not actually lost weight when in fact they are just retaining fluids. This is especially true for women if they are taking cleansing herbs and colon cleansing, which I recommend. Remember, muscle weighs more than fat.

Many years ago, when I was on one of my usual weight loss diets, I went to a restaurant and had a large salad with only greens. I was so proud of myself thinking, *Oh, boy, tomorrow when I get on the scale, it will really show some loss of weight, right?* The scale actually showed that I had gained three pounds. I was sick and despondent that whole day.

It ruined my day! This is what the scale does to your life. It ruled my life. Now I rarely get on a scale, maybe two times a year.

The most successful way of determining weight loss is by measuring your waist and measuring your hips, which will reveal the true results of your weight loss and fasting success. I have in my closet skinny girl's pants, the size I find ideal to measure my weight changes. This is my weight loss determination.

Percentages of Calories from Fat

Beef fat content	29%
Chicken (without skin and white)	23%
Certain salmon	50%
Broccoli	8%
Potato	1%
Beans	4%
Rice	1% to 5%

Obesity

Why are Americans overweight? I believe it is a combination of many factors. From my experience, how I finally got my weight down and kept it down for all these years was exercise plus eating God-made foods, nutrition, and periodic fasting. I believe it is not *how much* you eat, it is *what* you eat! It is interesting to note that overweight people are always craving the wrong foods: the foods that are making them fat in the first place. It becomes a vicious cycle. They buy vitamins and minerals that are getting only 1 percent assimilation because they are fortified with chemical "vitamins" that do the body no good.

These are the reasons I believe we are embarrassingly overweight, more than any other country in the world:

- Eating animal products
- Toxicity in our foods and environment, resulting in a heavily toxic body
- Chemicals we are putting into our bodies, produced by the food manufacturers, such as high-fructose corn syrup and MSG

- Processing of the foods we eat
- Lack of exercise
- Dehydration
- Refined sugars
- Too many enriched products, where all of the enzymes and nutrients have been removed
- Addictions to sugar products and animal products
- Toxins, poisons, herbicides, insecticides, carcinogens, free radicals—the list is endless—that have accumulated in our bodies, hindering us from losing weight and keeping fat on us
- Not enough fiber in our diet
- Not enough alkaline foods in our diet
- Genetically modified foods, which have had the nutrients removed
- Not drinking enough water
- Not enough nutrients

Some health practitioners believe obesity is caused by ongoing hunger. This is because food is depleted of nutrients. They are processed, canned, etc., so the body is not getting the nutrients it needs and continues to cry out, "I am hungry. Feed me."

Even when people are full, they are not truly nourished, so they continually have hunger. This is an epidemic: 50 percent of the American people have type 2 diabetes; 50 percent have a fatty liver. Dr. Amen discovered in a recent study: "brain scans show that the brain shrinks in overweight people."

A double-blind study was done, and one group of people was instructed to eat throughout the day, snacking throughout the day. The other group of people was instructed to eat only twice a day, not changing the contents of the food. At the end of that period of time, they discovered that the people who ate twice a day lost five pounds, while the people who ate throughout the day lost no weight at all.

People who eat animal-based diets have the highest amount of fat and toxins in their bodies. That is why you rarely see an overweight person who eats a strict plant-based diet. Americans are the fattest people on the planet. My estimation is that 80 percent of the American people are overweight. Just go to a Walmart, mall, grocery store, or bank, and count for yourself. By age sixty-five, we have stuffed over fifty tons of food in our body. When thin foreigners come here and embrace our standard diet, they begin to look like us: fat!

Suggestions for Weight Loss

1. Fast twenty-four hours one time each week. Be sensitive to the fact that when you start eating again, you could be ravenous. So be careful not to overeat!
2. Fast seven days one time every six months.
3. Eat no animal products. That includes eggs, dairy, fish, or chicken.
4. Snack on an apple a day.
5. Eat only God-made foods: fruits, vegetables, grains, legumes, raw nuts, and raw seeds. Remember more vegetables and fruits.
6. Exercise. Break out in a sweat five days a week for at least thirty minutes. If you have not recently exercised, start off with fast walking for thirty minutes and then build it up to some sort of cardio. I suggest Zumba.
7. Drink ten glasses of purified or distilled water every day (carry it with you everywhere you go).

8. Make a plan; you know two things for sure each day. You will go to the bathroom, and you will eat. Place dried fruit and/or raw nuts and seeds in the glove compartment of your vehicle. Know what you will be eating that day and have it readily available. Make a plan.

9. Use Himalayan salt for seasoning your food and lots of spices and herbs.

10. Eat only fibrous foods. Remember, fiber absorbs fat and toxins.

11. Use the palm of your hand as a guide. Your stomach is the size of your fist (or at least it is supposed to be). Eat foods that will fit on the palm of your hand, except for salads and vegetables. Eat all of the salad you want with raw sunflower seeds or raw pumpkin seeds. Those will make you feel full along with the salad. Add your dressing please.

12. Read labels! If it has chemicals in it or it is processed, do not eat it.

13. The bread to eat is two slices of the one mentioned in Ezekiel 4:9 or two non-GMO corn tortillas each day.

14. Do not get on the scale. To keep track of your weight loss, keep a tight pair of pants in your closet and use those as a guide. The scale will deceive you. At times, you can show a weight gain, even though you have been doing everything right. It could be water, menstrual cycle, etc.

15. Measure your waist and hips and remeasure in seven days. The slower you lose weight, the longer you keep it off!

16. Detox your body one time every six months and take cleansing herbs and colon cleanse. You can go to www.millanchessman.com or www.aonefastingretreat.com for help.

Plateau

Have you ever been on a weight loss program and losing weight quite successfully, then one day the weight simply stopped coming off? You try everything to jump-start the weight loss process to no avail. You try diet change, exercise change, and nothing works; no matter what you do, you just simply cannot drop another pound. So what happens is you can't meet your weight loss goal, and sometimes it can be only ten more pounds. This is a complaint I hear quite often, but I have good news for you: this problem is usually resolved through fasting. Sometimes, you can fast for three days, and, bam, the weight loss starts to proceed. That fasting could involve juices, Master Cleanse, or purified or distilled water.

Scale Is Your Enemy

You don't want to lose weight too fast. The slower you lose, the longer it stays off. Remember, muscle weighs more than fat, and the scale does not know the difference. The scale is an obsession. It is just a number and only one measure of progress and success. Don't rely on it. Weigh only every two to three weeks. High sodium retains fluids. In the summertime, you will weigh more as dehydration can cause fluid retention. Stress will cause you to weigh more, and studies show those that get less than seven hours sleep regularly are more likely to be obese. When we are tired, we are more likely to crave high-calorie foods. An examination of some ten thousand people on a three-year period found association between dehydration and obesity.

Exercise

I did no exercise of any kind until I turned fifty years old. I remember my son telling me, "Mother, you need to exercise if you want to lose weight." Finally, I did and have not stopped since. Now, I do Zumba six days a week and teach Zumba twice a week. Believe me, I am the oldest person in the class, and I break a sweat. Breaking a sweat is important. Some take a little longer to accomplish this than others. We have ninety-six million pores in our body. Exercise will create perspiration, which benefits the skin in becoming glowing and healthy and pulls out impurities.

Benefits of Sweating

1. Boosts endorphins
2. Enables detox
3. Lowers risk of kidney stones
4. Prevents colds and the flu
5. Zaps zits
6. Relieves stress
7. Kills bacteria and viruses
8. Improves blood flow

Exercise has helped me keep my weight down dramatically. Most people have poor muscle tone, and they are flabby, especially if they have been overweight and then lost weight. Exercise will change all that.

I want to add here that if you have a lot of weight to lose, please don't feel you have to start with a whole lot of exercise. First thing's first. I remember going to the gym and seeing overweight ladies doing extensive weights, and they just got bigger. They were not losing weight. This happened to me. I was doing very little cardio and trying to build muscle when I was overweight. I was frustrated because I felt like I looked bigger, which I probably did. Save lifting weights until you have obtained your normal weight. If you need to lose weight, then incorporate some cardio in your daily activities. Listen to your body, but do at least ten minutes a day of cardio, preferably dance.

A recent study in the *Journal of Applied Physiology* found that eating a low-carbohydrate meal after aerobic exercise enhances your insulin sensitivity. This is highly beneficial, since impaired insulin sensitivity, or insulin resistance, is the underlying cause of type 2 diabetes and a significant risk factor for other chronic diseases, such as heart disease. Consuming sugar within this post-exercise window will negatively affect both your insulin sensitivity and your human growth hormone (HGH) production.

Dancing Makes You Smarter

A twenty-one-year study of senior citizens by the Albert Einstein College of Medicine in New York City found that frequent dancing reduced the risk of dementia in seniors aged seventy-five years or older by 76 percent. It also found that reading reduced this risk by only 35 percent, doing crossword puzzles reduced it by 47 percent, and bicycling, swimming, or playing golf reduced the risk of dementia by 0 percent. Additionally, dancing has the ability to reduce stress and depression, increases energy and serotonin production, and improves overall flexibility, strength, balance, and endurance. Dancing strengthens bones and boosts cardiovascular health, increases mental capacity, and creates new neural paths. It tones the entire body, is fun, boosts heart health, helps de-stress, improves coordination, and makes you happy. Zumba burns six hundred to one thousand calories in one hour.

In the past, there has always been the trend to make people lie down and rest while they are fasting. The books all said: no exercise. Today, we have learned that is not always necessary. If you are feeling that you need to exercise while you are fasting, by all means, go for it. I just advise you not to push yourself or overexert yourself if you are feeling wiped out. If you are overweight and you are fasting, doing a little cardio will intensify the weight loss.

I want to add something *very important* here. One of the benefits of fasting you want to accomplish is to rid the body of carcinogens, impurities, toxins, poisons, etc., which assists in weight loss. This requires energy. This is the same energy you normally use to exert yourself, physically. If you push yourself to do cardio of any kind, you can slow down the detoxification of your body. When you rest during your fast, your body starts to dump these impurities more effectively that is what you want to accomplish. Some fasting counselors encourage exercise. I say listen to your body. After you complete the fast, then you can exercise all you want, but remember to listen to your body.

I remember not practicing what I preached one time. I went to the gym to do an aerobics class. Oh, my goodness, my body just ached, and I thought, *What am I doing here? I am fasting, and I should be home resting.* After thirty-six years of fasting experience, I feel qualified to give this advice.

CHAPTER 4

Cancer and Its Related Topics

Esther and her household fasted without water or food for three days then boldly and illegally entered into the king's presence to save her people and succeeded.

—Esther 4:16

Cancer

Charlotte Gerson states that cancer is "caused by nutrient deficiency and toxicity." There are literally thousands of people who have put their cancer into remission by switching to a plant-based diet. You want to search for the cause of cancer and not just treat the symptom. A lousy diet and the buildup of impurities resulting in a challenged immune system are the cause, and now you must do what is necessary to reverse it by eating a plant-based diet. Girls who start their menstrual cycle earlier in life have a higher risk of breast cancer, as well as other diseases and premature death. Girls in foreign countries that eat a plant-based diet start their cycle in much later years. Additionally, studies now show a correlation of abortions and breast cancer.

There was a four-year study done in which half of a group of women with cancer ate plant-based diets and the other half ate the standard American diet. Forty percent of the women that ate the animal-based diet had recurring cancer, yet not one woman on the plant-based diet had recurring cancer.

Cardiovascular diseases have claimed over one million lives in the United States, accounting for almost half of all deaths. Every thirty-three seconds, an American dies from cardiovascular disease. Heart disease and cancer are two consequences of an animal-based diet. Animal-based diets feed cancer; plant-based diets feed your immune system.

In 1961, President Nixon declared war on cancer, and yet today we have more cancer than ever before. It is a multibillion-dollar industry. A cancer treatment is considered a success if you live for five years. If one dies in the sixth year, it is still considered a success. This is something to think about. The cure for cancer is our immune system. Our immune system is weakened because of the animal-based diet, processed foods, chemicals, carcinogens, etc., in the standard American diet. Those eating a plant-based diet in other parts of the world have very little cancer.

You probably have heard as I have that black pepper is not good for you, but now recent studies find that black pepper has anticancer effects and is therefore good for you. Those who have had cancer were studied, and it was discovered that the more chamomile tea they drank, the more cancer cells dropped. It has been discovered that just eating oatmeal for breakfast has the ability to increase one's life span.

Twelve proven benefits of drinking coffee

1. Better work out and physical performance at the gym
2. Can help you burn fat
3. Contains essential nutrients
4. May lower your risk of type 2 diabetes
5. May protect you from Alzheimer's disease and dementia
6. May lower risk of Parkinson's disease
7. May protect your liver
8. Can fight depression and make you happier
9. May lower risk of certain types of cancer
10. Doesn't cause heart disease and may lower stroke risk
11. May help you live longer
12. Increases beneficial gut bacteria

Antioxidants

When you age, your body oxidizes, so eat foods with antioxidants. Antioxidants fight cancer and remove free radicals from the body which cause cancer. The amount of antioxidants you put into your body will determine how long you live. Dr. Michael

Greger states from his studies that the top antioxidant foods are cloves and cocoa powder. Vegetables with the highest antioxidants are red cabbage and artichokes; the fruit with the highest antioxidants are goji berries, acai berries, and blueberries.

The more color in vegetables, the more antioxidants they carry. Red onions are far healthier than yellow onions and white onions. The second top bean in the bean family for phytonutrient content are lentils. Tempeh is the highest in phytonutrient in the soy family, and edamame is second highest. Walnuts and pecans are the healthiest nut to eat. Dr. Michael Greger states that raw foods are not necessarily healthier; according to the most recent research, cooked vegetables as well as raw have nutritional benefits. Raisins can drop our bad cholesterol level by 13 percent. The better raisins are golden which have higher antioxidants than sun-dried raisins. Currants are the healthiest dried fruits to eat. Red leaf lettuce is healthier than green leaf lettuce and iceberg lettuce. Two cups of green tea each day will drop our stroke risk by 50 percent, and it can be beneficial in reducing the risk of obesity as well. Drink your tea cold; it has more antioxidants, and it is healthier for you. There are some studies that link the lack of friendly flora, *L. acidophilus* and *Bifidus*, to obesity.

Food

"Let medicine be your food and food be your medicine," stated Hippocrates, our first physician. Wouldn't it be great to pay our doctors for keeping us healthy, rather than bombarding us with prescription drugs that do not make us healthy but ultimately sicker and sicker? You can rid the body of diabetes and prevent it altogether by eating a strict plant-based diet. I am one of those people. I was diagnosed with borderline diabetes when I was thirty years old. My mother and father were both type 2 diabetics, and the doctor said that I would be a diabetic as well. Now, as a senior, I am not a diabetic.

Eating light meats does not help you to lose weight. The MD told me to eat fish and chicken. Chicken does not reduce your cholesterol levels. It has almost the same amount of cholesterol as beef. Sure, I would lose a pound or two, but I would get off the diet, and, boom! I'd put on weight again, plus more. More and more evidence shows that diabetes is a result of eating animal products, not sugar. Chicken, turkey, and eggs have cryptocides, a toxin that causes cancer. Read *Conquest of Cancer*, by Dr. Virginia Livingston, MD.

There is a protein in dairy that can trigger juvenile diabetes. As bad as dairy is for our bodies, most doctors still recommend milk every day. Remember: our nutritional guidelines and nutritional standards are set by politicians. They are in the pockets of the cattle and dairy industries as well as others. How many Americans do you know that do everything right yet die prematurely by following government guidelines? The average child is exposed to over ten thousand food messages on television every year, and so many are not true. I remember my daughter, Johnell, watching TV as a child, would call out to me. "Mommy, they are lying again on TV."

I have had clients, myself included, experience conflict, criticism, and attitude from others who do not understand anything about health and food choices. For example, I would be eating with friends and family and would choose not to eat the same unhealthy foods they were eating, such as animal products, fried foods, processed foods, etc. The attitude was: "Who do you think you are by not eating like me?" What some of my clients have chosen to do is simply say, "The doctor said I cannot eat that." That is the end of that conversation, and there is then peace.

Plant-based foods contain over one hundred thousand different disease-preventing nutrients. Chili peppers are very good for you. They prevent infections and gastric bleeding. They can also prevent cancer and have an anti-inflammatory role in the body. Cayenne is excellent for blood flow and prevention of varicose veins and heart attacks.

Dates are considered almost an ideal food and are very good for us. Date syrup is great for preventing diabetes. Dates and date syrup have no adverse effect on our blood glucose level, even large amounts. They also have phytonutrients. Eating a vegetarian diet boosts antiaging enzyme activity by 300 percent.

Let's discuss nuts. Eating nuts will not make you fat. Always remember your stomach is supposed to be the size of your fist, so grab a handful of nuts and enjoy. Nuts can suppress cancer growth. Walnuts and almonds will decrease inflammation, pistachios are high in antioxidants, and pecans are one of the highest foods in antioxidants. A handful of pistachios could reduce bad cholesterol. Eating peanut butter reduces the risk of suffering heart attacks by 50 percent. Hurray for this, because I love peanut butter and have always heard that it is bad for your digestion and not a healthy food to eat. Now new studies are showing just the opposite. I believe that roasted nuts can be problematic. Why? Studies have shown that eating nuts will actually help you lose weight, but roasting nuts can destroy nutrients and enzymes and, therefore, can cause weight gain.

Listen and highlight this: your tastes *can* change. This I promise. Give yourself twenty-one days eating God-made natural foods such as fruits, veggies, grains, legumes, and raw nuts and seeds. Eat nothing else. These are called transition foods. Don't look back. Watch as your taste buds change and your waistline gets smaller. But I want to warn you: if you sneak a bite of cheese, or any food other than those listed above, you will never have victory. I truly believe that. It must be all or nothing! Then if you try to eat something that is unhealthy, it will taste unpleasant.

Benefits of a Plant-Based Diet

- Bowel regularity
- Weight loss
- More energy
- Better mental clarity
- Beautiful skin
- Slows down the aging process
- Increased libido
- Less sickness and disease
- No more food cravings
- Stronger immune system

The following is a list of foods and their nutritional benefits:

Food	Benefits
Apple	Protects your heart, prevents constipation, blocks diarrhea, improves lung capacity, cushions joints

Apricot	Combats cancer, controls blood pressure, saves your eyesight, shields against Alzheimer's, slows aging process
Artichoke	Aids digestion, lowers cholesterol, protects your heart, stabilizes blood sugar, guards against liver disease
Avocado	Battles diabetes, lowers cholesterol, helps stop strokes, controls blood pressure, smoothens skin
Banana	Protects your heart, quiets a cough, strengthens bones, controls blood pressure, blocks diarrhea
Bean	Prevents constipation, helps hemorrhoids, lowers cholesterol, combats cancer, stabilizes blood sugar
Beet	Controls blood pressure, combats cancer, strengthens bones, protects your heart

Blueberry	Combats cancer, protects your heart, stabilizes blood sugar, boosts memory, prevents constipation
Broccoli	Strengthens bones, saves eyesight, combats cancer, protects your heart, controls blood pressure
Cabbage	Combats cancer, prevents constipation, promotes weight loss, protects your heart, helps hemorrhoids
Cantaloupe	Saves eyesight, controls blood pressure, lowers cholesterol, combats cancer, supports immune system
Carrot	Saves eyesight, protects your heart, prevents constipation, combats cancer, promotes weight loss
Cauliflower	Protects against prostate cancer, combats breast cancer, strengthens bones, banishes bruises, guards against heart disease

Cherry	Protects your heart, combats cancer, ends insomnia, slows aging process, shields against Alzheimer's
Chestnut	Promotes weight loss, protects your heart, lowers cholesterol, combats cancer, controls blood pressure
Chili pepper	Aids digestion, soothes sore throat, clears sinuses, combats cancer, boosts immune system
Fig	Promotes weight loss, helps stops strokes, lowers cholesterol, combats cancer, controls blood pressure
Flax	Aids digestion, battles diabetes, protects your heart, improves mental health, boots immune system
Garlic	Lowers cholesterol, controls blood pressure, combats cancer, kills bacteria, fights fungus

Grapefruit	Protects about heart attacks, promotes weight loss, helps stop strokes, combats prostate cancer, lowers cholesterol
Grape	Saves eyesight, conquers kidney stones, combats cancer, enhances blood flow, protects your heart
Green tea	Combats cancer, protects your heart, helps stop strokes, promotes weight loss, kills bacteria
Honey	Heals wounds, aids digestion, guards against ulcers, increases energy, fights allergies
Lemon	Combats cancer, protects your heart, controls blood pressure, smoothens skin, stops scurvy
Lime	Combats cancer, protects your heart, controls blood pressure, smoothens skin, stops scurvy

Mango	Combats cancer, boosts memory, regulates thyroid, aids digestion, shields against Alzheimer's
Mushroom	Controls blood pressure, lowers cholesterol, kills bacteria, combats cancer, strengthens bones
Oat	Lowers cholesterol, combats cancer, battles diabetes, prevents constipation, smoothens skin
Olive oil	Protects your heart, promotes weight loss, combats cancer, battles diabetes, smoothens skin
Onion	Reduces risk of heart attack, combats cancer, kills bacteria, lowers cholesterol, fights fungus
Orange	Supports immune systems, combats cancer, protects your heart, strengthens respiration
Peach	Prevents constipation, combats cancer, helps stop strokes, aids digestion, helps hemorrhoids

Peanut	Protects against heart disease, promotes weight loss, combats prostate cancer, lowers cholesterol
Pineapple	Strengthens bones, relieves colds, aids digestion, dissolves warts, blocks diarrhea
Prune	Slows aging process, prevents constipation, boosts memory, lowers cholesterol, protects against heart disease
Rice	Protects your heart, battles diabetes, conquers kidney stones, combats cancer, helps stop strokes
Strawberry	Combats cancer, protects your heart, boosts memory, calms stress
Sweet potato	Saves your eyesight, lifts mood, combats cancer, strengthens bones
Tomato	Protects prostate, combats cancer, lowers cholesterol, protects your heart

Walnut	Lowers cholesterol, combats cancer, boosts memory, lifts mood, protects against heart disease
Water	Promotes weight loss, combats cancer, conquers kidney stones, smoothens skin
Watermelon	Protects prostate, promotes weight loss, lowers cholesterol, helps stop strokes, controls blood pressure
Wheat germ	Combats colon cancer, prevents constipation, lowers cholesterol, helps stop strokes, improves digestion
Wheat bran	Combats colon cancer, prevents constipation, lowers cholesterol, helps stop strokes, improves digestion

Prescription Drugs

Doctors tend to treat the symptoms of a bad diet with medications. It is a lot easier to tell a person to take a pill than it is to tell them to change their diet. We are a very "want it now" society. An MD friend told me that MDs get two hours of nutrition the whole eight years of medical school. An average of twelve new prescriptions are written per person every year. Almost 243,000 people are hospitalized each year because of reactions to prescription drugs. Medical errors are the third leading cause of death in United States, causing at least 250,000 deaths every year. There are four hundred deaths a day from side effects of prescription drugs, and 163,000 people suffer drug induced memory loss or impaired thinking.

I believe the reason people are living longer today than before is because today, people are given prescription drugs to band aid health issues especially pain. For example, I know a man who is seventy years old and has painful arthritis, so painful sometimes he can hardly walk. He goes to the MD periodically for cortisone steroid injections, and pain is gone and he feels great again. Studies show that patients that received steroid injections lost more cartilage than those who got saline. This is exactly the opposite of what patients and their doctors would want to happen. What a terrible side effect. This is one example why I believe people live longer today but sicker than in years past.

In 1962, I was pregnant with my first child. Because I had always struggled with obesity, I asked my MD to give me something to take so that I would not put on extra weight. I was very young and very ignorant. You won't believe this, but he wrote a prescription for amphetamines. *Speed.* So I took them the last five months of my pregnancy. Can you imagine! Speed while I was pregnant. Thank God, I had a beautiful healthy baby who, to this day, is lovely and healthy.

Contraindications

"Can I fast if I am taking prescriptions?" People ask me that all the time. I tell them: it is your body; it is your decision and no one else's. I cannot tell anyone not to take prescriptions. I will say this: I have had many people come to my fasting retreat and decide not to take their prescriptions and have succeeded in obtaining optimum health.

Here is a quote from Dr. Paavo Airola, who wrote *How to Keep Slim, Healthy and Young with Juice Fasting*: "As a rule, a complete withdrawal of all drugs is advised during a fast. However, in certain conditions when drugs have been used for a long time and a certain body dependence has built up, withdrawal of drugs should be gradual, and the effect of withdrawal carefully supervised by a doctor."

This is very controversial, and the opinions of one fasting expert will be different from another. I will tell you of my experience. I had numerous people who stayed at my fasting retreat and were type 2 diabetics taking insulin. Each day of the stay, their blood sugar levels were tested. On the seventh day, their blood sugar was normal. I have had many clients taking prescription drugs for depression who decided to abstain from the drugs during a fast and went away with no more depression. I recommend you counsel with a knowledgeable health practitioner on this subject before you begin an extensive fast.

I lectured a few years back at the Cancer Control Society and was asked to participate at a symposium consisting of various medical doctors and health practitioners. I gave my talk to this audience and spoke of how people with type 2 diabetes have benefited and put their disease in remission through fasting. I have had many of these people come to my retreat. In the medical arena, you always hear "people with diabetes must never go without food." Where that opinion came from, I do not know. But at my fasting retreat, that is simply not the case. After my talk, one MD stood up and just lit into me, scolding me and reprimanding me for depriving someone that was a diabetic of food. There is so much misinformation about fasting. Remember, practically all diseases can recover through fasting, even when one is underweight.

CHAPTER 5

Nutrients

Jesus fasted forty days when in the wilderness, which was the beginning of His three-year ministry.

—Matthew 4:12

Enzymes

Enzymes are a very important part of your diet. You normally have enzymes in your body, which I compare to having a bank account: you have a bank account of enzymes, and it's like having funds in a bank account. As you live your life and eat unhealthy foods, you remove from your bank account the enzymes to digest those unhealthy foods. Generally, the more of your enzyme bank account you deplete, the faster you age, the sooner you die, and you become prone to obesity, sickness, and disease. Eat foods that are loaded with enzymes. The more raw foods you eat, the more enzymes those foods have for you to digest and to nourish your body. Eat a salad or a green smoothie every day. Talk about nutrition! You can feel the difference in energy, weight loss, and optimum health!

Indigestion and heartburn are caused by deficiency of stomach enzymes. Most people over age forty have some deficiency of digestive enzymes, which are important to assimilate the nutrients in our foods. I recommend you take phytonutrients while you are fasting. These are green powder, consisting of many fruits and vegetables, that is loaded with nutrients and assimilate into your body instantly. Most vitamins are sold as fractionated chemicals and do not help; they are fortified. They are synthetic, but you can't fool the body. The best nutrients you can get for your body are in "organic" foods, especially greens, fruits, raw nuts, seeds, legumes, grains, and fresh juices or smoothies. A low-fat diet can make heart patients sick. Glucosamine taken alone can make arthritis worse because it can leach from the body other essential bone health nutrients. Remember one thing about fasting: our hydrochloric acid increases so that we can better assimilate our nutrients. Fasting will help the body to assimilate the nutrients such as vitamins and minerals and all other essential nutrients that are necessary for optimum health.

The Hunger Hormones	
Leptin	Suppresses the appetite, maintains energy balance, regulates ghrelin
Ghrelin	Increases appetite, signals hunger to the brain, regulates body weight
How to control the hunger hormones	• Eat fewer fatty foods, especially in the days before a fast • Fast twenty-fours one time a week • Eat more vegetables and less refined sugar

Vitamins

Vitamin B12 is very important for you, and those who eat a vegan diet should take it. I recommend "B Supreme" brand, due to the absorption and effectiveness of this product. I take it every night when I climb into bed, break it into pieces, and place them under my tongue for absorption. Let me tell you my story: we were going to India and were told to get vaccinated for malaria because of its prevalence there. Mosquitoes would travel for miles to get to my husband, so we were concerned. We were told by my daughter, Roxanne, to take the B vitamins for two weeks before our trip, and the mosquitoes would not bother us. We did, and while staying in a hotel-converted palace which had very high ceilings, we could see lots of mosquitoes on the ceiling. This was the big test. We turned off the lights, and sure enough, here they came. Buzzing around our faces, *but* we did not get one bite. Not one! All of the other folks we traveled with got bitten, but we did not.

The story does not end there. A year later, we traveled to Guatemala and Honduras and again were told to get malaria shots. We took a different brand of the "B" vitamins, and this time, we got bitten by the mosquitoes, so quality is important. My daughter, Johnell, told me recently that when she went down to Cabo San Lucas, she got many mosquito bites. She forgot to take the "B Supreme." A year ago, when she went to El Salvador, which is known for malaria, she diligently took the "B Supreme" for two weeks before the trip and did not get one mosquito bite.

What this product will also do is help you gain control of food addictions such as sugar and animal products. Yes, one can be addicted to animal products. The B12 from animal products has very little absorption, and animal products destroy the "B" vitamins in the body. Vitamin B deficiency can cause depression, weight gain, and hair color change and increases addiction to foods. When you attempt to stop eating animal products, you will get weak, have cravings, and will feel lethargy. That is simply your body detoxing. The "B Supreme" helps with these addictions. Also, you will find that you will begin to lose weight. Children who are vegans need to be sure to take their B12 vitamins. "B Supreme" is tasty, and the children will love it! There are so many benefits to good quality B vitamins. It eases stress, anxiety, and depression, aids memory, relieves

PMS, reduces heart disease risk, builds up immune system, and provides more energy, as well as better skin, hair, and eyes.

Basking in Vitamin D

- It is thought that up to 90 percent of US senior citizens may be vitamin D deficient, along with 70 percent of the American public.
- African Americans and other dark-skinned people and those living in northern latitudes make significantly less vitamin D than other groups. One nationwide study of women revealed that almost half of the African-American women of childbearing age might be vitamin D deficient.
- Sixty percent of patients with type 2 diabetes have vitamin D deficiency.
- Studies show very low levels of vitamin D among women, children, and the elderly.
- Winter, when sun exposure is at its lowest, is the time of year when you need to be most concerned about the amount of vitamin D you are receiving, as your vitamin D levels can drop by up to 50 percent in the winter. Of course,

if you have the tendency to spend the summer months indoors, out of the sun, or you only go outside with sunscreen on, then you would need to be concerned during the summer months as well.

Vitamin D deficiency doubles your risk of cancer. Researchers now agree that this epidemic of a wide variety of cancers may be due to widespread vitamin D deficiency, which is caused in large part because of sun avoidance.

The cancers most strongly linked to low levels of vitamin D are:

- Breast cancer
- Colon cancer
- Lung cancer
- Prostate cancer

Vitamin D has a protective effect against cancer in several ways, including:

- Increasing the destruction of mutated cells (which, if allowed to replicate, could lead to cancer)

- Reducing the spread and reproduction of cancer cell
- Causing cells to become differentiated (cancer cells often *lack* differentiation)
- Reducing the growth of new blood vessels from preexisting ones, which is a step in the transition of dormant tumors turning cancerous

If you take oral vitamin D, make sure you take the correct type. There is one warning you need to be aware of if you choose to use an oral vitamin D supplement: there are two types, natural and synthetic. The natural one is D3 (cholecalciferol), which is the same vitamin D your body makes when exposed to sunshine. The synthetic one is vitamin D2.

Recent studies. Do not take vitamin E supplements alone, as you will live a shorter life, according to recent studies; it is harmful to the body. What many people, including health professionals, fail to realize is your cells have two receptors for vitamin A, for every one vitamin D receptor. There is a vitally important relationship between vitamin A and vitamin D. If you receive too much vitamin D, vitamin A will help protect you from an excess. This is a crucial concept to understand, as many individuals will take this new information regarding vitamin D, and start to take massive doses, thinking that this would be a good thing. You simply were not designed to ingest your vitamin D but rather to absorb it from the sun on your skin.

Sunlight. The vitamin D that you get from sunshine helps your body to make that supplement. Studies have shown that getting fifteen minutes of sun every day will cut your risk of getting breast cancer by 50 percent. The following is a quote by Dr. Mercola: "You need an average of at least ten to fifteen minutes of sunlight every day to prevent cancer." A breakthrough study which was recently published demonstrated just how important getting regular exposure to sunlight is for you. Regularly spending even relatively short intervals of only ten to fifteen minutes in the sunlight allows your body to produce vitamin D, and having adequate vitamin D levels can drastically reduce your risk of cancer. The researchers, from the Moore's Cancer Center at the University of California, San Diego (UCSD), estimated that by increasing vitamin D3 levels, particularly in countries north of the equator, 250,000 cases of colorectal cancer and 350,000 cases of breast cancer could be prevented worldwide. In all, that amounts to 600,000 cases of breast and colorectal cancer prevented, including close to 150,000 in the United States alone. This is an unprecedented study because it's the first to take satellite measurements of sunshine and cloud cover in the same countries where blood serum levels of vitamin D3 had also been taken.

In addition to preventing about six hundred thousand cases of cancer each year, the researchers concluded that increasing the intake of vitamin D3 throughout the world could easily prevent diseases that would otherwise claim close to one million lives each year. Yes, it's true; this flies in the face of most public health statements and "expert" physicians' recommendations to stay *out* of the sun. Sun exposure, they say, can lead not only to skin cancer but also to premature aging of the skin (wrinkles) and cataracts. It is vital for you to understand, right here and now, that the dangers of sun exposure have been greatly exaggerated and the benefits highly underestimated. I am not exaggerating here when I tell you the very life of you, your family, and your friends hangs in the balance unless you understand the truth about this issue. It is more than worth your time to analyze your belief about this topic because if you choose wrong, you could easily leave this world earlier.

I believe that the evidence is very clear; you are not nearly as likely to develop deadly skin cancer as you have been led to believe, and the benefits you will receive from normalizing your vitamin D levels continue to be documented daily in scientific literature.

Why sunlight is healthy. How do the benefits of sunlight so vastly outweigh the risks? Vitamin D, the sunshine vitamin, is entirely different from any other vitamin you have heard of because it is not really a vitamin at all but a prohormone that your body actually produces from cholesterol. Because it is a prohormone, it influences your entire body—receptors that respond to the vitamin have been found in almost every type of human cell, from your brain to your bones. Regular exposure to UVB from sunlight (which in turn increases your vitamin D levels) reduces your risk of the following diseases:

- Sixteen types of internal cancers
- Diabetes
- Heart disease

- Hypertension
- Multiple sclerosis
- Osteoporosis
- Psoriasis
- Rickets
- Schizophrenia
- Tuberculosis
- Myopathy

Your simple cure for most coughs and colds. Instead of relying on potentially dangerous and ineffective over-the-counter remedies for cough and colds, your solution may simply be to get outside and have more sun exposure on as much uncovered skin as possible. This is because vitamin D has also been found to cause your immune system T cells—the cells that destroy damaged and infected cells—to change shape and migrate to the uppermost layer of your skin. This may also help explain why vitamin D has such a protective effect against skin cancer in particular. Magnesium contributes to the assimilation of vitamin D.

Aside from helping to prevent cancer, vitamin D is also excellent for your heart and can increase your body's production of naturally occurring antimicrobial peptides, which destroy the cell walls of viruses and bacteria. Sunlight was used as early as a century before the discovery of antibiotics as an effective tuberculosis cure. Tuberculosis (TB) is a potentially deadly disease that is spread by air-borne bacteria, which settle in the lungs and result in long-term infections. TB is currently responsible for more deaths worldwide than any other single infectious disease. Auguste Rollier began using sun-light therapy to treat TB in Switzerland in 1903, with such success that, over the course of the next forty years, his methods were adopted by hospitals worldwide. Of the 2,167 patients who were under his care for tuberculosis following World War I, 1,746 completely recovered their health, an aston-ishing number for the time, with the only failures being those who were already in the most advanced stage of the disease. Studies have also shown that metabolizing vitamin D can restrict the growth of tuberculosis within cells. In one study, Indonesian scientists found that treating tuberculosis patients with ten thousand units of vitamin D daily (instead of the much smaller amount usually advocated by conventional medicine) led to a cure rate of 100 percent—everyone in the study was cured. Quite impressive indeed!

Tuberculosis is not the only disease documented to be influenced by vitamin D. Sunlight has also been shown to be effective against anthrax, cholera, *E. coli*, dysentery, influenza, staphylococcus, streptococcus, and other illnesses. There are also a number of physiological mechanisms triggered by vitamin D production—through sunlight exposure—that act to fight heart disease, according to the *British Journal of Nutrition*, including:

- An increase in the body's natural anti-inflammatory cytokines
- The suppression of vascular calcification
- The inhibition of vascular smooth muscle growth

Recent studies have shown vitamin D is more effective in preventing the flu than the vaccine.

Optimizing your omega-3s to prevent skin cancer. If you consume the standard American diet, you are probably not getting enough omega-3s in your diet. This is unfortunate for a number of reasons, but in the context of sunlight, omega-3 fats will dramatically cut down your risk of skin cancer. Further, your ratio of omega-3 to omega-6 fats is a very important key to lowering your cancer risk. As a general rule of thumb, most people in the United States are consuming far too many omega-6 fats (found in vegetable oils like corn, soy, canola, safflower, and sunflower oil) and too few omega-3 fats (found in flaxseed oil, walnut oil, olive oil, and chia seed). Additionally, mothers that took omega-3s during pregnancy found their children had better vision at two months old, significantly better problem-solving at nine months old, and significantly smarter at four years old when compared to those who did not ingest omega-3.

CHAPTER 6

A Closer Look at Soy Products vs. Animal Products

Moses fasted for 40 days and wrote the 10 commandments.

—Exodus 34:28

Dairy Products

Dairy products are the number one source of inflammation and weight gain. Inflammation can lead to painful arthritis. Have you ever seen the hands of an older person? They are crooked, and the joints are all swollen. This is the outcome of arthritis, and dairy is one of the greatest causes of this condition. I did a test on myself: for three days, I ate chunks of cheese, the pasteurized, homogenized kind. On day four, I could feel the pain of arthritis, and my joints were visibly swollen. It was awful! The only thing I did differently was eat these chunks of cheese. I then stopped eating the cheese, and the next day, the pain disappeared. I don't eat pasteurized, homogenized cheese; instead, I will buy vegan cheese. "Follow Your Heart is a delicious brand." It is delicious, and once in a while, I buy raw goats' cheese. It does not give me this condition. Of course, moderation is the key.

The average person consumes thirty pounds of cheese per year. Cheese is one of the biggest contributors to obesity. The cheese you purchase in the main grocery stores is pasteurized and homogenized. That means all of the nutrients and enzymes have been destroyed. When you eat this cheese, it plays havoc on the body. It creates excess mucus in the stomach and small intestines. Excess mucus hinders the body from assimilating nutrients because it coats the stomach. Cheese can also be addictive. It has addictive properties such as traces of casomorphins. It causes severe constipation, acne, cancer, especially breast and prostate cancer, hormonal disturbances, and hypertension. It provides higher risk for type 1 and 2 diabetes and arthritis, more than any other food. The cholesterol content is worse than it is in meat. It is very unhealthy. When you remove dairy, headaches go away, digestive problems improve, and arthritis diminishes.

The number one source of clogged arteries is saturated fat coming from dairy. It is one of the top allergy causes in the food industry. What we get in dairy is lactose, butter fat, pesticides, antibiotics that are GMO, bovine hormones, and cytocides. There is pus in every glass of milk. The dairy council claims it's okay because they pasteurize it. Pasteurization kills the bacteria, so it doesn't matter how infected the udders of the cows are, according to the dairy council. Many studies have shown that there is significantly more acne among dairy-eating teenagers. I believe cutting out dairy products can help alleviate the phenomenon.

Most Americans suffer from excess mucous and allergies, today more than ever before. What causes so much mucous in our bodies? I believe it is the kinds of foods that we are ingesting, especially dairy. When we eat animal foods, which the body was never meant to digest, the body starts to protect itself and coats the stomach and small intestines with mucous. This excess mucous hinders the body from assimilating nutrients that are so vital for optimal health. Then comes a time when we get a cold or runny nose. This happens when mucous has built up and now needs to expel from the body. In my opinion, this is not a bad thing; it is good to get it out of your body. But what is even more beneficial is to stop the accumulation to begin with.

The Dietary Guidelines Advisory Committee warns people who choose not to consume cow's milk that they risk malnutrition by stating, "Those who choose not to consume milk and milk products (cheese, yogurt, etc.) should include other foods in the diet that contain the nutrients provided by the milk and milk products group: protein, calcium, potassium, magnesium, vitamin D and vitamin A." Remember, spinach and other veggies have plenty of protein; as long as you eat a whole, plant-based diet, you will get more than enough in the above-listed nutrients. The only vitamin that is very important to add is vitamin B12. The Dietary Guidelines Advisory Committee recognizes that dairy foods that are loaded with saturated fats which cause clogging of the arteries. Remember, these foods have no fiber, and you need fiber to flush out fat from the fat cells, which is so very important for weight loss. That cellulite you see is simply fat and toxins in the cells. Fasting removes both.

Eating Animal Products

Human beings have the digestive system of an herbivore. We have twenty to twenty-two feet of small intestines and five to five and a half feet of large intestines. The animal that eats plants also has a long digestive system. The carnivore has a short digestive system. As it says in the Bible, God gave us plants to eat (Genesis 1:29). Prior to the flood, it is recorded that man lived as long as 969 years. Man ate plants, and there was no recorded case of sickness and disease. After the flood, because everything was under water, man resorted to eating animals. He acquired an addiction to eating animals, and the aroma of roasting meat was enticing. The life span then dropped to 150 years, and sickness and diseases were recorded.

From 1970 to today, there has been one new disease every year. We are putting into our bodies what we were never created to eat. The damage animal products do to the body includes kidney stones, liver and kidney damage, heart disease, cancer, osteoporosis, arthritis, removal of serotonin from the brain, and added carcinogens. Serotonin is needed to keep a person calm, composed, and mentally stable. Studies have shown vegetarians display less depression, anger, mood swings, mental illness, etc. than those who eat animal products, because of the serotonin that stays in the brain. Animal products pull out the serotonin that is necessary for us to have tranquility and peace. This is also due to an inflammation of the brain caused by eating animal products. Every other client I see suffers or has suffered from depression and panic attacks. These are just a few diseases caused by eating animals.

Americans eat seven thousand animals in their lifetime. That results in tons of feces in our water, earth, and environment. It is estimated that an individual consumes approximately 225 pounds of meat every year. Today's kids especially get affected by meat addiction and are in worse shape health-wise than all of the kids of past generations in the history of this great country!

The benefits of a meatless diet are many which include reduced risk of heart disease, loss of excess body weight, reduced cancer risk, dropped blood pressure, reversed diabetes, and lowered risk of Alzheimer's disease. The animal food industry has conducted studies that say animal foods are not detrimental to our health. They then collect billions in subsidies from our government and all of the profits. All this while, Americans get sicker and bigger. Compared to people in other countries, Americans are morbidly obese. It is a shocking and embarrassing phenomenon. The types of flora in the digestive system are related to body weight and weight gain. There is a belief that possibly vegetarians are thinner because of the type of bacteria in their digestive system. Remember that animal products cause putrefactive bacteria that kill the friendly bacteria that we need. Also, our body odor is more pleasant if we have the good bacteria in our bodies.

It is becoming more evident that consuming meat regularly increases our risk for diabetes. Women who eat animal products have the highest levels of estrogen in their blood stream. Also, milk blocks the natural phytonutrients in chocolate. Dairy milk is produced from lactating cows, which is why we have higher estrogen hormone levels in our bodies. This increases breast cancer and prostate cancer. This does not happen with organic soy milk.

I never saw a man with breasts in years past; now, many men have breasts. The cause is the dominant female hormones, like estrogen, are found now in dairy products. Certain toxic chemicals accumulate in the fat tissues; therefore, a vegan's body is less polluted than those of omnivores.

Studies have shown that early maturation in American teens is a direct result of drinking cow's milk and eating dairy. This is a direct result of the hormones that are given to cows to hasten maturation of cattle, which has the same effect on young boys and girls. Recently, my grandson turned thirteen years old, and I was absolutely shocked to see the numerous girls he invited to his birthday party whose physical appearances were dramatically mature beyond their years; these twelve- and thirteen-year-olds had bodies like full-grown women. Early puberty results in a shorter life span. Kids who eat animal products reach puberty one year earlier than kids who eat a plant-based diet.

All animal products are now being fed genetically modified food, consisting of corn, grains, and nonorganic soy. They are also given hormones to make them grow very quickly and grow bigger, antibiotics, and growth stimulators, in addition to other drugs. These animals are placed in a very unhealthy environment; many are fed dead carcasses of other animals, making them carnivores when they really are herbivores.

Steroids are given to cows to "beef" up their muscles faster, just like athletes take steroids to build up their muscles. It has been shown that if an athlete eats a lot of meat and then is tested, he can be accused of taking steroids. Parasites, blood vessels, nerves, and cartilage can be found in beef, and the meat content in each hamburger that was purchased in five fast food eating places was only 2–14 percent. What was also found in these hamburgers was ammonia. The reason they found so much ammonia was because it is being used to kill the bacteria found in animal products. They actually inject the beef with ammonia to kill the bacteria. There was a story released about a prison in Georgia that sent all the meat back because of the strong smell of the ammonia in the meat. It wasn't even good enough for the prisoners.

Fifty pounds of all kinds of fish were analyzed in New York according to *Vegetarian Times Magazine*. They discovered that 85 percent had DDT and 80 percent had mercury, which kills brain cells and causes cancer. Forty percent of the fish contained human fecal matter. The fish with the least of these toxins were the fish with fins and scales.

Two thirds of fish tested came up positive for parasites. In fish fillets, they found Benadryl, cortisone, Zoloft, and Prozac, as well as other drugs. Fish oil has so many toxins in it that it is recommended to eat flax and algae to get your DHA omegas. Recent studies show no benefit in taking fish oil. Flaxseed oil is healthier and has more nutrients in it, and it is wonderful for elimination as well. Where do the fish get their omegas from? They get it from the sea plants, such as microalgae. Where did the cows get their calcium? They got it from plants. Even if fish oil is distilled, studies have shown it is not safe or beneficial. Polychlorinated biphenyls (PCBs), a toxin, can promote obesity and heart disease. Industrial chemical pollutants are also related to obesity and are found in the human body. They disrupt our metabolism and predispose us to obesity. These toxins, called obesogens, are found mostly in animal products such as fish, which is top of the list. One single serving of canned tuna is equivalent to one hundred vaccines in terms of the mercury content. That would be about a half a can of tuna.

Most recent studies are taken from Dr. Michael Greger's MD research. A Harvard Study followed twenty thousand doctors who ate eggs for twenty years and discovered that just eating one egg a day had higher mortality rate. The more eggs we eat, the shorter we may live. Alfalfa sprouts should not be eaten because of the *Salmonella* epidemic, but eggs are two thousand times more contaminated with salmonella, and yet nothing is ever mentioned about that in the media. Eggs are among the highest in cholesterol, which contributes to heart disease. Half an egg eaten a day raises your risk of certain cancers. Animal products have cholesterol, while plants have no cholesterol. Eliminating animal products from the diet opens up the arteries, and the body actually gets younger.

I believe the members of the Dietary Guidelines Advisory Committee know the truth about the role that animal products play in causing the vast majority of chronic diseases that afflict Americans today (heart disease, type 2 diabetes, obesity, osteoporosis, and cancer, all of which are mentioned in their report). I believe they also know the solution to the health problems Americans face, since they recommend taking steps to "shift food intake pattern to a more plant-based diet that emphasizes vegetables, cooked dry beans and peas, fruits, whole grains, nuts, and seeds." They should have stopped right there, but they didn't. Instead, they continued on with the following recommendations: "In addition, increase the intake of seafood, and fat-free and low-fat milk and milk products, and consume only moderate amounts of lean meats, poultry, and eggs." With just this one industry-friendly sentence, the consumer is given permission by the Dietary Guidelines Advisory Committee to continue eating animal foods (albeit in moderation) that have caused our nation's current health crisis.

Parasites

Here is one of many reasons I don't eat animal products. Long before I knew anything about health, we had a freezer packed full of meat in the little storage room of our home, all kinds of meat, seafood, chicken, you name it. My son unplugged the freezer to plug in the iron to iron something and forgot to plug the freezer back in, and we took a two-week vacation immediately after. We had locked our home up tight as a drum. When we came back from vacation two weeks later and opened the garage door where the storage room was connected, the smell was the most putrid I'd ever smelled. We then opened up the storage room where the freezer was, and that room was filled with flies. The smell was horrible! When we opened up the freezer where all the rotten meat was, there were thousands of maggots all over the frozen rotten meat. I ask you: where did those maggots come from? How did they get into the freezer? You and I know that they were already in the frozen meat that we were going to eat. This is how unhealthy meat is for our bodies.

I remember, when I was in high school, my mother took red snapper fish from our freezer to prepare for our dinner. She placed it on our kitchen counter and marinated it. When she returned around 5:00 p.m. to cook it, there were worms crawling all over it. Fish is the wormiest food to eat.

People who eat sushi and come to my retreat almost always expel parasites. The reason is because we provide three powerful parasite products that are taken three times each day at my retreat. One of the most dramatic episodes I remember was a lady who was slim; she ate very healthy, and yet she kept coming back to my retreat because she complained of digestive issues. She came three separate weeks, about three to four months apart, and did colon hydrotherapy daily, totaling twenty-one colon therapy sessions. On the last day of her stay, she passed a three-foot worm in the colonic tube. I have done over thirty thousand colonics and *never* have seen a worm that long. We were both speechless. After that, she never came back. She recovered from her digestive issues which I presume were caused by the giant worm. There are so many instances that I have seen worms and parasites come out of people's bodies, too many to mention.

Soy Products

There are no negative impacts made on the body when organic soy is consumed, yet soy has gotten a bad rap. Women who eat soy cut their risk of ovarian cancer in half. Studies show men who drank soy milk provide protective measures against prostate cancer. See nutritionfacts.org for more information on these results.

There is a lot of controversy about eating soy. I say, "If it is good enough for the Japanese who have been eating soy for five thousand years, it is good enough for me." Japanese are the longest living people in the entire world. Women in Japan have less breast cancer than women anywhere else in the world. I eat organic soy; it is a great transitional food for those who are trying to get off eating animal products. They make so many meat substitutes from soy. I eat a lot of tempeh and organic tofu. They make great sandwiches, prepared properly. Eating soy can cut our diabetes risk by 50 percent, according to the most recent research. Just make sure the soy is organic, if you can. Chances are that if it is not organic it is GMO.

Soy products in recent studies have been shown to drop bad cholesterol by 14 percent, and it is excellent for weight loss. Not only does soy prevent cancer, but soy cuts the risk by 50 percent of those that have cancer. Women who had cancer and ate soy cut their risk of dying by 50 percent. This is from the most recent studies. Women with breast cancer who eat soy actually live longer! Americans who increased tofu consumption were significantly associated with decreased breast cancer risk.

Benefits of organic soy:

- Reduces symptoms of allergic asthma
- Strengthens bones
- Protects nerve cells
- Inhibits various cancer developments
- Lowers body fat
- Improves insulin responses to blood sugar
- Lowers cholesterol
- Stops plaque from developing in blood vessels
- Slows aging process
- Keeps weight in control

The University of Illinois study found improved kidney function and elevated levels of good cholesterol when ingesting organic soy. A study in Brazil compared skim milk to soy milk. In six weeks, bad cholesterol went down, and good cholesterol went up, which was exactly the reverse of what happened drinking cow's milk. The study concluded that the high consumption of organic whole soy foods was the main reason the elderly Okinawans have 80 percent fewer heart attacks and low rates of various cancers. Good soy products are organic tofu, tempeh, edamame, miso, shoyu soy sauce. Soy baby formula is consumed a lot here in the United States, but what is so sad is that these babies are more than likely drinking GMO soy. This is a terrible health hazard. People complain they are allergic to soy and probably are because they are eating GMO soy. Remember, 95 percent of the soy grown in the United States is genetically modified. See chapter 9 for more about GMOs.

CHAPTER 7

Check Out Those Ingredients

Ezra humbly fasted and prayed for protection against the enemy—and received victory!

—Ezra 8:21–23

Refined White Sugar

Refined white sugar causes weight problems, irritability, depression, cravings, and addictions. It destroys "B" vitamins, which are desperately needed to improve mood and regulate weight. This kind of sugar creates free radicals, which ultimately cause cancer, causes mood swings, and uses up our important enzymes. It leaches calcium from our bones, hair, and nails and redeposits it to joints, which then can cause arthritis, backaches, bursitis, etc. It also affects our pancreas and makes us tired and lethargic. Refined white sugar causes mental decline leading to diseases of the brain. When the brain goes, that is it! Who wants to live if we cannot communicate or think for ourselves? Excess refined sugar causes clogged arteries, which can lead to strokes. Have you ever seen someone who had a stroke? It is horrible! The average teenager eats one hundred pounds of refined white sugar a year. Refined sugar has been whitened by a chemical that causes cancer.

Artificial sweeteners include acesulfame K, aspartame, neotame, saccharin, and sucralose, which are all approved for use in the United States. All of these sweeteners are chemically manufactured molecules, molecules that do not exist in nature. Splenda or aspartame converts to formaldehyde and destroys brain cells, whereas NutraSweet causes brain damage and depression. Other artificial sweeteners include Fructose and Equal, which cause migraines, PMS, depression, Alzheimer's, allergies, and fibromyalgia.

Some good sugars to use are as follows: xylitol, natural maple syrup (my favorite), barley malt, raw sugar, raw honey, birch sugar, stevia, and date sugar. A study was done on two groups of individuals. One group was given regular sodas (Pepsi and Cokes), and the other group was given diet sodas for one week. They discovered that the group given the diet sodas actually *gained* weight. I believe this weight gain was caused by all of the chemicals designed to make one addicted.

Food Additives

Some food additives are worse than others. Here's a list of the top food additives to avoid:

1. Artificial sweeteners

Aspartame (E951), more popularly known as NutraSweet and Equal, is found in foods labeled "diet" or "sugar-free." Aspartame is so harmful that leading scientists have asked the FDA to pull it from the market. Aspartame is believed to be carcinogenic and accounts for more reports of adverse reactions than all other foods and food additives combined. It produces neurotoxic effects such as dizziness, headaches, mental confusion, migraines, and seizures. Avoid it especially if you suffer from asthma, rhinitis (including hay fever), or urticaria (hives). Acesulfame K, a relatively new artificial sweetener found in baking goods, gum, and gelatin, has not been thoroughly tested and has been linked to kidney tumors.

Commonly found in the following: diet or sugar-free products (sodas, Jell-O and other gelatins, desserts, gum, drink mixes like Kool-Aid, baking goods, table top sweeteners, cereal, breath mints, pudding, iced tea, chewable vitamins, and toothpaste).

2. High-fructose corn syrup

High-fructose corn syrup (HFCS) is a highly refined artificial sweetener which has become the number one source of calories in America. It is found in almost all processed foods. HFCS packs on the pounds faster than any other ingredient, increases your LDL ("bad cholesterol") levels, and contributes to the development of diabetes and tissue damage, among other harmful effects. Almost all foods have this chemical except organic. Why? To make you addicted to it. If you want to lose weight, you must start reading labels and stay away from this chemical.

"When fructose is consumed, it appears to behave more like fat with respect to the hormones involved in body weight regulation," explains Peter Havel, associate professor of nutrition at the University of California. "Fructose doesn't stimulate insulin secretion. It doesn't increase leptin production or suppress production of ghrelin. That suggests that consuming a lot of fructose, like consuming too much fat, could contribute to weight gain."

Another study by researchers at the Children's Hospital Boston found that every additional eight-ounce soft drink in a day increased school kids' risk of being obese by 60 percent, due to the high-fructose corn syrup and other chemicals. This popular sweetener is your enemy when it comes to your health and weight loss. It can be addictive, and it is put in processed foods to make you want to eat more.

Commonly found in the following: most processed foods, breads, candy, flavored yogurts, salad dressings, canned vegetables, and cereals.

3. Monosodium glutamate (MSG/E621)

MSG is an amino acid used as a flavor enhancer in soups, salad dressings, chips, frozen entrees, and many restaurant foods. MSG is known as an excitotoxin, a substance which overexcites cells to the point of damage or death. Studies show that regular consumption of MSG may result in adverse side effects, including depression, disorientation, eye damage, fatigue, headaches, and obesity. MSG affects the neurological pathways of the brain and disengages the "I'm full" function, which explains the effects of weight gain.

Fast food restaurants add MSG to their foods. Why? To make you addicted. In many studies around the world, scientists were creating overweight mice by injecting them with MSG. MSG is in almost all processed foods except organic.

If you want to lose weight, you must read the labels very carefully. There are over twenty-five names on labels that mean MSG, such as "flavors," which makes reading labels all the more difficult. Health professionals agree that MSG and high-fructose corn syrup are chemicals that are deliberately put into our foods to make us addicted and eat more. I believe this is one of the reasons we see such obesity in the United States.

One of the biggest abusers of MSG is restaurant fried chicken. Now you know why you can't stop eating the coating on the skin. What do you think their secret spice is? Yes, MSG. Now there is a link between MSG and migraines, autism, Alzheimer's, and diabetes. "Not only is MSG scientifically proven to cause obesity, it is an addictive substance." Since its introduction into the American food supply fifty years ago, MSG has been added in larger and larger doses to the prepackaged meals such as soups, snacks, and fast foods which we are tempted to eat every day. "Increased numbers of people with obesity have become rampant since then."

Commonly found in the following: Chinese food, many snacks, chips, cookies, seasonings, most Campbell's Soup products, frozen dinners, and lunch meats. There are twenty-eight other names put in as ingredients which mean MSG. Here are twenty-one of them:

- Glutamic acid
- Glutamate
- Monosodium glutamate

- Monopotassium glutamate
- Calcium glutamate
- Monoammonium glutamate
- Magnesium glutamate
- Natrium glutamate
- Yeast extract
- Anything hydrolyzed
- Hydrolyzed protein
- Calcium caseinate
- Sodium caseinate
- Yeast food
- Yeast nutrient
- Autolyzed yeast
- Textured protein
- Soy protein isolate
- Whey protein isolate
- Vetsin
- Ajinomoto

4. Trans Fat

Trans fat is used to enhance and extend the shelf life of food products and is among the most dangerous substances that you can consume. Numerous studies show that trans fat increases LDL ("bad cholesterol") levels while decreasing HDL ("good cholesterol"). It increases the risk of heart attacks, heart disease, and strokes and contributes to increased inflammation, diabetes, and other health problems. Trans-fatty acids in margarine cause more than thirty thousand Americans to die of heart disease every year.

Commonly found in the following: margarine, chips and crackers, baked goods, and fast foods. It is originated from synthetic and animal products.

5. Common food dyes

Studies show that artificial colorings, which are found in soda, fruit juices, and salad dressings, may contribute to behavioral problems in children and lead to a significant reduction in IQ. Animal studies have linked other food colorings to watch out for:

- Blue #1 and Blue #2 (E-133)
    - Banned in Norway, Finland, and France. May cause chromosomal damage.
        - *Found in:* candy, cereal, soft drinks, sports drinks, and pet foods

- Red dye # 3 (also Red #40, a more current dye) (E124)
  - Banned in 1990, after eight years of debate, from use in many foods and cosmetics. This dye continues to be on the market until supplies run out! Has been proven to cause thyroid cancer and chromosomal damage in laboratory animals and may also interfere with brain-nerve transmission.
- *Found in:* fruit cocktail, maraschino cherries, cherry pie mix, ice cream, candy, bakery products, and more!
  - Yellow #6 (E110) and yellow tartrazine (E102)
    - Banned in Norway and Sweden. Increases the number of kidney and adrenal gland tumors in laboratory animals and may cause chromosomal damage.
- *Found in:* American cheese, macaroni and cheese, candy and carbonated beverages, lemonade, and more.

6. Sodium sulfite (E221)

This is a preservative used in wine making and other processed foods. According to the FDA, approximately one in one hundred people is sensitive to sulfites in food. The majority of these individuals are asthmatic, suggesting a link between asthma and sulfites. Individuals who are sulfite sensitive may experience headaches, breathing problems, and rashes. In severe cases, sulfites can actually cause death by closing down the airway altogether, leading to cardiac arrest.

Commonly found in the following: Wine and dried fruit

7. Sodium nitrate

A common preservative usually added to processed meats like bacon, ham, hot dogs, and corned beef. Studies have linked sodium nitrate to various types of cancer.

Commonly found in the following: cured meats such as bacon and luncheon meat, hot dogs, and anything smoked.

8. BHA and BHT (E320)

Butylated hydroxyanisole (BHA) and butylated hydroxytoluene (BHT) are common preservatives which keep food from changing color, changing flavor, or becoming rancid. They affect the neurological system of the brain, alter behavior, and have the potential to cause cancer. BHA and BHT are oxidants, which form cancer-causing reactive compounds in your body.

Commonly found in the following: potato chips, chewing gum, cereal, frozen sausages, enriched rice, lard, shortening, candy, Jell-O, and vegetable oils.

9. Sulfur dioxide (E220)

Sulfur additives are toxic, and in the United States, the Food and Drug Administration has prohibited their use on raw fruit and vegetables. Adverse reactions include bronchial problems particularly in those prone to asthma, hypotension (low blood pressure), flushing, tingling sensations, or anaphylactic shock. It also destroys vitamins B1 and E. Sulfur additives are not recommended for consumption by children. The International Labor

Organization says to avoid E220 if you suffer from conjunctivitis, bronchitis, emphysema, bronchial asthma, or cardiovascular disease.

Commonly found in the following: beers, soft drinks, dried fruit, juices, cordials, wine, vinegar, and potato products.

10. Potassium bromate

An additive used to increase volume in some white flour, breads, and rolls, potassium bromate is known to cause cancer in animals. Even small amounts in bread can create problems for humans.

Commonly found in breads

Chemicals

I read a report which stated that sports drinks can dissolve the teeth. Chemotherapy is a form of mustard gas that was used in World War I. The cause of *Candida albicans* is primarily the result of chemicals we are ingesting. Chemicals slow down digestion and cause gas, bloating, toxins, and constipation. Our bodies were never intended to ingest chemicals, yet we see them in all processed foods, except organic. The preservatives, BHT, BHA, and TBHQ, are made from petroleum, which is meant for our car, not our stomachs. Artificial colors cause allergic reactions. A standard lemon meringue pie has eighteen preservatives. Just remember: "Thou shall not eat anything that thou cannot pronounce."

Salt

A new study published in the *American Journal of Hypertension* questions the benefits of a low-salt diet, *USA Today* reports. Although earlier findings show that cutting back on sodium reduces blood pressure, they also reveal that it causes a significant rise in cholesterol and triglycerides. Additionally, this diet produced higher levels of rennin, an enzyme that regulates blood pressure, along with increased levels of noradrenalin and adrenaline, hormones that influence blood pressure and heart rate. While it is not clear at the present time that these changes would lead to more heart attacks and strokes, the results cast some doubt on the healthfulness of the low-salt diet.

The release of this research ignited the expression of much dissenting opinion among members of the American medical community, who contend that the results should be taken "with a grain of salt." Lawrence Appel, of the John Hopkins School of Public Health, states the results were unreliable, due to the small size and short duration of the study, *CNN Health* relays. A spokesperson for the American Heart Association opines that it would not be detrimental to cut back on salt, since the American diet is very high in this mineral. Although the American Heart Association recommends a diet with 1,500 mg of sodium per day, the typical American consumes over twice this amount. But should people really be concerned about their salt intake? Not according to the study's author, Niels Gradual, of Copenhagen University Hospital in Denmark, who states that generally people should not worry about it. Gradual told Reuters that based on the total evidence he does not see a benefit of reducing salt consumption in the general populace.

This new research follows another recent European study that shows a low-salt diet was linked to an increased risk of heart-related deaths. Furthermore, this same investigation found that higher sodium levels were not associated with a higher incidence of blood pressure problems or complications from heart disease in those who are otherwise healthy. However, until more studies examine the long-term consequences of the possible negative effects of the low-salt diet, American doctors will not likely accept the results of the recent European studies as being valid. I eat salt but only Himalayan salt, as it has all minerals, and I use it generously. It is all natural.

Exploding the Myth of the Low-Salt Diet
(Don't Risk Your Health Even One More Day by Cutting Down on Salt)

Dear Newsmax Friend,

I don't salt my food anymore. At least, not with regular old table salt. Yet I'm not on a low-salt diet, either. I use plenty of salt to spice up my food, just not the toxic kind that is in most kitchens. That's because of what I've discovered recently from Dr. David Brownstein, the medical editor of our latest *Newsmax* publication. When you ask him about the low-salt diet recommended by most conventional doctors, even the American Heart Association and the American Diabetes Association, he says: "Phooey!"

And here's just one reason *why* he says it…

For nearly everyone, a low-salt diet does *not* lower blood pressure. It's true. Even in those individuals with high blood pressure, the lowering effect is quite modest at best. Still, Dr. Brownstein will tell you that he learned in medical school the traditional party line that salt = hypertension (high blood pressure). But he began researching the therapeutic use of salt when many of his patients did poorly on a low-salt diet. Plus, many of them didn't remain on the diet because it made their food tasteless and dull.

Heart Disease Deaths Four Times Higher with Low-Salt Intake

The Journal of the American Medical Association (JAMA) is also changing their tune about salt intake. Natural health professionals have long valued salt for cardiovascular balance among other benefits.

Studies show that people with greater salt intake are the ones more likely to avoid hypertension, heart disease, and death. Doctors never really could explain why they believed lower salt intake would improve heart health. But don't expect conventional doctors to sing the praises of salt any time soon.

Reputations of doctors and high-ranking government officials could be harmed if the truth were acknowledged. The waste of massive amounts of the public's money in promoting lower salt intake would betray the political health of elected officials. In that world, the actual health of the people carries little weight. Salt reduction is being enforced in the food industry. Schools are reducing salt in lunches.

Humans have understood the value of salt since we have existed. It was traded among the earliest communities on earth—likely back in the times of cave dwelling. We use expressions like "salt of the earth" because of the recognition of its value.

Dr. David Brownstein, board-certified physician, has lectured internationally to physicians and others about his success in using natural hormones and nutritional and holistic therapies in his practice. And when he began practicing a more holistic form of medicine, Dr. Brownstein was surprised to find that most of his patients were actually deficient in minerals. He made an interesting connection to the use of refined salt and this deficiency.

Refined or regular table salt has *no* minerals. Patients with chronic illness are often more mineral deficient than those who are comparatively well. Minerals such as magnesium, sodium, chloride, and potassium are vital for life. After researching various types of salt, Dr. Brownstein found the solution in the form of unrefined salt. Unlike refined table salt, *unrefined* salt contains over eighty essential minerals. He started recommending it to his patients, and a funny thing happened, when his patients began using unrefined salt as part of their holistic treatment regimen:

- Their mineral deficits improved.

- Those with high blood pressure began to see their numbers decrease.
- He noted that patients with immune and hormonal problems also began to get better.

How could this happen? *Without salt, life itself would not be possible.*

Salt is as important to life as oxygen and water. In fact, salt and water work together to do important work in your body, including stimulating your metabolism, helping you detoxify, and making sure your nerves, hormones, and immune system function properly. Yet the food industry has sold you a "bill of goods" on refined salt for the same reason they refine other products like sugar, flour, and oils to *maximize their profits*. For one thing, the refining process, which eliminates all of salt's life-sustaining properties, ensures that it won't go rancid. That salt can sit on the shelf forever, with no expiration date. This saves the food industry a heck of a lot of money. And then there's marketing. Salt manufacturers have found that an "all-white" product appears cleaner and more appealing to you, the consumer.

But Everyone Says Salt Is Bad for You…

Despite the fact that scientific research does not support the claims for low salt diets, even the US Food and Drug Administration (FDA) are getting into the act. They are now considering regulating salt as a dangerous substance! The salt controversy is so full of half-truths and downright lies that Dr. Brownstein decided to tackle it head-on in the second issue of his *Newsmax* newsletter *Natural Way to Health*.

Rubbing Salt into the Wound

By not having an adequate salt intake, you are exposing your body to a real danger. You see, we humans put a great value to the sense of taste. Now, the four major tastes are salty, sweet, bitter, and sour. The latter two are not really desirable, and by eliminating salt, we are left only with sweet. So here's what's happening: in our effort to cut out the salt, we willingly or unwillingly take in more sweets (in other words, refined sugar). And here is the real kicker: our body has a way of getting rid of the extra salt (taste your skin if you don't believe me), but extra sugar assists in converting fat, which poses the biggest risk to our cardiovascular health. Thus, placing too much emphasis on reducing salt detracts from far more dangerous substances in food, which is very unfortunate.

Choose Your Salt Wisely

There are many types of salt. Unfortunately, the table salt we regularly consume is not healthy. There is an ocean of difference (literally) between table salt and sea salt. Sea salt contains many minerals like magnesium, which enables nerve transmission and muscle contraction, induces relaxation, relieves constipation, promotes bone formation, and reduces blood pressure and heart disease. Not only does table salt exclude these minerals, but it also contains various unhealthy additives—aluminum, dextrose, and even bleaching agents. Sea salt is alkalizing to the body, whereas table salt is acid forming. The modern diet is already overly acidic, and sea salt helps to restore balance due to its mineral content. Sea salt also tastes saltier than table salt, so less is needed.

Indeed, restricting sodium may actually have an adverse effect. *Moderation* is the key, not strict salt reduction. But a word of caution: most products branded as sea salt are actually refined and inferior. A simple rule of thumb to recognize unrefined sea salt is "if it's white, it's not right." Unrefined sea salt is typically grayish, or it can have a red or black hue. Personally, I use Himalayan salt to my heart's content, since it is loaded with almost all minerals. So pass the saltshaker, please!

Wonderfully Alkaline

pH Alkaline Strips

Alkaline strips arc a simple at home test. It will test the pH of your body to tell you if you are alkaline or acidic. You want to show alkaline. Ideally, should read 6.8 to 7.2. Generally, if you are alkaline, you will not get sick as easily or gain weight, and you probably will be losing weight if you are overweight. I test my pH almost every morning around 6:00 or 6:30 a.m. I call it "Pee and See." I say this is my body telling me if I am healthy or not. These little strips are very inexpensive and easy to use; I advise you to start doing this on your own as well. In fact, when someone says to me, "Oh, Millan, I can't hug you, I have a cold," etc., I say, "Don't worry, my immune system is strong, and there is no concern that I will contract your illness."

Upon rising, take the strips with you to your bathroom and simply urinate on the strip. It is best if you do this on the first urine elimination after the sun rises so that you can have a more accurate reading. I personally have the strips sitting next to my toilet. This is my doctor at home because this shows me what my body needs from me that day. If I show acidic, usually from eating too many beans, corn tortillas, and rice, I will immediately add alkaline foods to my diet. I am very careful about this. You can email me, and I will send it to you with my alkaline/acid food chart. You should ideally eat 80 percent alkaline foods and 20 percent acid foods. If you show acid (a yellow color on the strip), then you could be gaining weight, and your immune system is weak, making you vulnerable to sickness and disease. Simply get back to eating more alkaline foods. If you are fasting, your pH will read acidic. That is to be expected. Your body is in a detox state, and for the first four days of your fast, it will read acidic. The ancient Anasazi Indians lived to an average life span of thirty-eight years old. Their diet was exclusively beans, corn, venison, and squash, all acid foods. Is there a correlation? I think so.

CHAPTER 8

Cleanse and Hydrate Will Exhilarate

Fasting is necessary for overcoming some demonic powers.

—Mark 9:29

What Are Colonics?

Colonics, lymphatic cleansing, ion foot spas, cleansing herbs, and the like are hot topics in the health industry today for good reason. The foods we are eating hardly have any fiber and nutrients, since there is so much processing of our foods. The average American is walking around with between five and fifteen pounds of waste in their body. Look around and see all of the pot bellies. It's no wonder people are cleansing. Dr. Norman Walker, who lived to be over one hundred years old, stated "death and disease begins in the colon."

What are colonics? It is a procedure which gently cleanses the intestines of waste that builds up from a non-fiber diet, mostly animal products, which have no fiber. It's like getting a bath inside the body. The therapist is a gentle, caring individual who has knowledge in this field. Be sure she or he is qualified with proper training. I have been an instructor and member of I-ACT (International Association of Colon Therapists) since 1994. This is an organization with strict colon therapy safety guidelines. Cleansing herbs taken just before the colonic provide a more successful cleanse. Most colon hydrotherapy equipment have a fluorescent lit view tube where one can see the results of a cleanse.

One gentleman, Richard Smith, took his blood pressure before his colonic, and it read 171/102. After his colonic therapy, he took it again, and it read 151/88. That's awesome! Another client whose face was half paralyzed from a stroke and was unable to smile on that side of her face, did a series of a ten-cleanse program, and afterward, she was able to smile on the paralyzed side as well. Agent Orange was dumped on the American soldiers during the Vietnam war, and a very sick client who was one of those soldiers did a cleanse program, and you could see all of the Agent Orange coming out of his body during the colonic. He then totally recovered after thirty years of suffering.

If you are worried about the experience of getting a colonic, don't be. Talk to your colonic therapist prior to a cleansing, and ask them any questions that may come to mind. Here is what I tell most people: it's not painful, embarrassing, or offensive. Everything is contained in the closed system making it a very pleasant, comfortable experience. After your procedure, you get that same exhilarated feeling you have after you take a bath. You feel cleansed!

Colon Cleansing

Some people in the fasting industry do not advocate colonics. That just does not make sense to me. Remember, when we are fasting, the intent is to flush out carcinogens, toxins, poisons, and free radicals. What better way to do that than incorporating colon hydrotherapy? It just makes good sense. When you are fasting, your digestive system is not functioning, it is resting. Because the average American is carrying five to fifteen pounds of waste in his digestive system, wouldn't it make sense to wash it out with a colonic?

The testimonials are absolutely mind-boggling. In the thirty-six years I have been in the health industry and supervising fasting clients, I have found colon cleansing, and cleansing herbs, along with a fast, produces better results, and you can see with your own eyes the sludge, sewage, etc. come out of your body! One picture is worth a thousand words. I passionately advocate colonics or enemas when you are fasting.

The difference between and enema and colonic is as follows: The water in an enema just reaches the sigmoid (lower part of the colon) to remove waste, whereas in a professional colonic, the water removes waste all the way to the beginning of the colon, which is five feet long. If a person takes cleansing herbs and does an enema, he or she will still get outstanding results. When you fast for weight loss, you get better results in the loss of the fat if you take the cleansing herbs and cleanse the colon. If you are going to go through all of the effort to fast, you might as well do what works best, right?

My Suggestions for Enemas

When you do an enema, you should do a good forty-five-minute enema. Lie on the floor and put filtered water with one-fourth cup olive oil and two tablespoons of lemon juice into the enema container. Insert the speculum (lubricated) into the rectum, unclamp the water, and as soon as you feel pressure, clamp the nozzle closed and allow the water to soak in the bowel. Once the pressure has subsided, put a little more water into the colon and repeat. Do this for about fifteen minutes, unless of course you really feel you need to sit on the toilet. Then sit on the toilet and release the water and waste. Repeat the process again as before for a total of forty-five minutes. Do this each day during your fast and take cleansing herbs. Don't do an enema without taking the cleansing herbs. When you do a colonic or enema, you are intensifying the cleansing process with better success. There are toxins in the fat cells, and you want toxins and fat released out of your body.

Cleansing herbs reduce your appetite big time MDs did colonics before the 1950s. Today, MDs will state that colon hydrotherapy can be habit forming, can perforate the bowel, or that it washes out the friendly flora. In all of my research, I have never found this to be the case. I have administered over thirty thousand colonics and have never had someone tell me they could not go to the bathroom without a colonic or enema. Just the opposite is the case. The colon muscle peristalsis works well, and the constipation is eliminated most of the time. When you change your diet to eat plant-based foods, you will have very healthy bowel movements every day! The colon therapy will wash out some of your electrolytes (minerals), but I recommend taking good quality minerals. You can order this from my website. Studies have been done to prove the friendly flora naturally multiplies when the colon gets cleaned out. Read my book, *Cleanse Internally to Become Younger*, for more information on cleansing.

Probiotics

There is a lot of discussion over taking probiotics when you are fasting. I personally don't think it's that important, and I will tell you why: a study was done in a naturopathic university where they took a group of people, tested the levels of probiotics in their bodies, and were told not to change their diets for a three-month period. During that three-month period, a series of colonics were administered. After the three-month period, they tested their levels of probiotics again and discovered that they had more friendly flora in their systems than before the colonics. Ideally, you should have 80 percent friendly flora and 20 percent coliform bacteria. Because of the incorrect and unhealthy diet, we have just the reverse, 80 percent coliform bacteria and 20 percent probiotic bacteria. Animal produces putrefactive bacteria which destroys the good bacteria.

I maintain that when you do colon hydrotherapy at my fasting retreat, you are giving the body an opportunity to increase its friendly flora. With the wisdom and knowledge that you have acquired at the fasting retreat, you will go home, and, with your healthy new eating plan, you will continue to have a high number of friendly flora in your body.

Water

The root cause of so many diseases is dehydration, simply put: lack of water. Our brain is 85 percent saltwater. The body is 75 percent water. Studies show 75 percent of the American people are dehydrated, and in 37 percent of Americans, the thirst mechanism is so weak that it is often mistaken for hunger. A study from the University of Washington has shown that one glass of water will shut down midnight hunger in almost 100 percent of dieters. This lack of water is the main reason for afternoon fatigue. A mere 2 percent drop in body water can trigger fuzzy short-term memory, trouble with basic math, and difficulty focusing on the computer screen or on a printed page. Drinking eight glasses of water a day decreases the risk of colon cancer by 45 percent, plus it can slash the risk of breast cancer by 79 percent and one is 50 percent less likely to develop bladder cancer according to recent research. I cannot overemphasize the importance of drinking at least two liters of water each day.

At my age, I consider myself extremely healthy. I exercise six times a week doing cardio, eat plant-based foods, fast, and detox periodically. Ten years ago, I started getting an intense pain near my left hip bone. In my thirties and forties, I remember when I would drive the eight-hour trip to my home town of Monterey, California, once a month, I would get that pain in that same area while driving that distance. I would get out of my car and stretch my legs, and the pain would subside. Then the same pain returned and was close to unbearable. If I sat for any length of time and stood up I would limp and thought, *Oh my goodness, I think I might become a cripple.* This went on for about six months. My family was concerned about me, so I went to an MD, a chiropractor, and a naturopath doctor and got no relief. I then watched a documentary on salt and water. At that time, I was drinking only one liter of water each day thinking that would be sufficient. The doctor in the documentary said if you want to get rid of pain, drink at least two liters of water each day. I then drank two and a half liters of water each day, and, lo and behold, on the third day, the pain was *gone* and has not returned. It was a miracle! I have not had any pain since and now that has been ten years.

These are the benefits of drinking two liters of water a day:

It curbs the appetite, hydrates the body, gives you more energy, helps break down nutrients in food, helps you lose weight, gives you lovely skin, and helps to overcome mental disorders, such as depression. It will lift your mood, gives you more mental clarity, and you will feel better. It will flush out the toxins, poisons, free radicals, and carcinogens and can stop most pain. Water is beneficial to hormone activity, bowel elimination, and prevention of water retention, believe it or not. Being dehydrated will release calcium from the bones. People will not even realize they are dehydrated because they don't feel thirsty and their mouth is not dry. Those are not the only signs of lack of water. Drinking water at the correct time maximizes its effectiveness on the human body.

- *Two glasses of water after waking up* helps activate internal organs.
- *One glass of hot water thirty minutes before a meal* helps digestion.
- *One glass of water before taking a bath* helps lower blood pressure.
- *One glass of water before going to bed* helps avoid stroke or heart attack.

The best water to drink is purified or distilled water. The authors of all the books that have been written on water are all advocates of distilled water. People will say that distilled water is not good because it flushes out your minerals, but that is only a half-truth. Distilled water flushes out inorganic minerals such as calcium deposits that are a detriment to your body.

"Organic minerals are very vital in keeping us alive and well. If we were cast away on an uninhabited island where nothing was growing, we would starve to death," Paul Bragg explains. "Years ago, I was on an expedition to China when one part of the country was suffering from drought and famine. I saw with my own eyes poor, starving people heating earth and eating it for want of food. They died horrible deaths because they could not get one bit of nourishment from the inorganic minerals of the earth."

These inorganic minerals can cause gallstones, liver stones, kidney stones, or acid crystals in different parts of the body, including veins, arteries, and joints. Distilled water does not remove the organic minerals that your body needs to sustain itself. I have been drinking distilled water for forty years.

In his book, *Miracle of Fasting*, Paul Bragg mentioned one of his experiences doing a thirty-day distilled water fast. On day twenty-one, he urinated, and a burning sensation occurred. Because he was a chemist, he knew he was passing something. He took that urine to the laboratory for examination and discovered he had passed ample amount of DDE, a derivative of DDT. It took twenty-one days for that toxin to be released out of his body. Imagine, had he stopped his water fast on day twenty, he would not have released that toxin.

CHAPTER 9

Toxic Cleanup by Fasting

David fasted one day in mourning the death of King Saul.

—2 Samuel 1:12

Toxins

A blood and urine study conducted on people at the Mount Sinai School of Medicine yields the following disturbing facts: 62 percent linked to brain and nervous system; toxicity was present; fifty-eight chemicals that are known to interfere with the hormone systems were present; fifty-five chemicals linked to cancer were present in their bodies; and fifty-three chemicals that are toxic to the immune system were also found, including band PCBs and DDT.

Additionally, ABC News reported the following alarming details: babies born from July to August 2007 were found to have one hundred industrial chemicals in their umbilical cord blood, including PCBs, fire retardants, mercury, etc. Over two hundred million tons of potentially dangerous pollutants have been released into our atmosphere. Three thousand toxic chemicals have been ingested into our bodies. We are ingesting one pound of food additives per person every year. In New York, there are roughly sixty tons of airborne toxins that fall monthly on each square mile. Fortunately, when we fast, we are removing these toxins that we inhale from our bodies.

Toxins to be concerned about are mercury, aluminum, cadmium, lead, arsenic, nickel, and uranium. Mercury accumulates in the brain, nervous system, and heart, as well as other parts of the body, according to studies. It is one of the deadliest substances known to man. It can cause memory loss, depression, tremors, heart attacks, anemia, etc. Mercury is used in dental fillings, and there is enough mercury in one dental filling to cause illness and brain malfunction.

In *The Miracle of Fasting*, Paul Bragg describes the result of one of his fasts: "I was at my family's old homestead in Virginia. On about the seventh day of a ten-day fast, I was out in a canoe on the river leisurely enjoying the sunshine and fresh air when suddenly, without warning, I doubled up with stomach cramps. I thought I would never be able to stand the pain! With great effort I got ashore and then it happened. I had a terrific bowel evacuation! At the end of this evacuation, I felt a heavy, cool sensation in my rectum and passed 1/3 cup of quicksilver (mercury) from the toxic Calomel that I took in my childhood."

The metals most commonly found in Alzheimer's patients are aluminum and mercury. The average person will consume over three pounds of aluminum in their lifetime, which destroys brain cells. The biggest source of aluminum getting into the body is deodorant. Never buy deodorant that has aluminum in it. Read labels on everything that goes into your body. Aluminum foil and pots and pans are a way of getting into the body as well. It is estimated that we eat one-third teaspoon of mercury, one teaspoon of lead, and one teaspoon of nickel in our lifetime. Fluoride consumption is also harmful to the brain, especially for children, whose brains are still developing. Additionally, fluoride causes arthritis, is toxic to the kidneys and the thyroid, and weakens bones.

There are new warnings about excessive Agent Orange toxin in baby formula and breast milk. This Agent Orange toxin is so widespread that babies are now born with toxic levels. It hides in animal proteins, including infant formula and breast milk, and is linked to numerous serious health problems. Now, the EPA is reviewing its safe limits. Agent Orange is the toxin that was dumped on the foliage in Vietnam to prevent the enemy from hiding. When it was dumped, it fell on our soldiers, and they also became toxic as a result.

Alloxan is the poison that is used to produce diabetes in normal rats, and yet it is added to white flour. Alloxan creates enormous amounts of free radicals and directly interacts with aspartame to produce multi-organ damage and advanced aging.

Genetically Modified or Genetically Engineered Foods

Genetically engineered foods cause disease with long-term effects. Rats given GE foods develop stomach lesions, smaller brains, and damaged immune systems. Studies on rats given GE foods also showed antisocial and fearful behavior. GE foods cause allergies, toxins, and lack nutrients. They are hazardous, and yet no safety studies are required on GE foods. GE foods are banned in Europe. They are known to cause birth problems. Many allergies to soy are due to the fact that the soy is genetically engineered. It can even damage DNA. Children eating GE foods are more susceptible to toxins and nutrition problems. Processed foods are usually GE foods. Ninety-five percent of soy, cotton, corn, and canola grown in the United States are GE. The pesticide that is GE in foods goes into a human and causes disease, damaged immune system, precancerous cells, and atrophy of the liver.

Now, all animals that we consume, except organic, are fed with GE food. GE foods leave genes behind in the body. These genes can jump from the GE food to gut bacteria and can create new diseases resistant to antibiotics. The gene produces the pesticide transferring to the gut bacteria. Now, we have a gene inside our gut bacteria, producing pesticides factories. Taken from *Vegetarian Times* in an article: "Something Fishy About My Sundae":

> *There is certain low-fat ice cream that has GE substance known as ice structuring protein (ISP) derived from the conger eel. These proteins allow low calorie/low fat ice cream to stay as creamy as full fat varieties when refrozen. ISP does not appear on the labels and there is no regulation in the US that requires foods and ingredients to be labeled as GE.*

Organic Foods

These foods are okay to buy commercial if you cannot find them organic: asparagus, avocados, broccoli, Brussels sprouts, cauliflower, cabbage, eggplant, garlic, onions (all varieties), rhubarb, sweet potatoes, and zucchini.

However, be sure to buy the following foods organic: celery, carrots, cucumbers, green beans, potatoes, spinach, winter squash, bell peppers, tomatoes, and beets.

A number of years ago, a client shared with me about her management and operation of a rest home for seniors who had health issues and were simply waiting to die. They were brought in by family members in wheelchairs and walkers and needed special care. She said they would sit and simply stare into space.

She began feeding them a solely plant-based diet. Veggies, fruits, healthy grains, legumes, brown rice, and nuts and seeds, all prepared from scratch. For refreshment, they drank only water. In three months, these folks were walking on their own with no assistance, speaking with each other, and had better clarity of mind. When their children came to visit, they were totally amazed to see such improvement with their family members. They would say: "I cannot believe the difference in my mother."

Recent Diseases and the Brain

People will say to me, "How do you explain that people are living longer today than they did back in the early 1900s?" Today, the average life span is somewhere in the late seventies, and back then, the global life span was thirty-one years old. I say yes, we are living longer today than we did back then; however, we are living longer, sicker, with no brain function. Do you want to grow to be an old, sick woman or man? I certainly don't. I want to live as a healthy senior with the ability to share love, wisdom, and service to others and to be an active grandmother and great grandmother.

Every sixty-seven seconds, somebody is diagnosed with Alzheimer's in the United States. Do you have any idea of what a horrible disease this is? An Alzheimer's patient cannot recognize his loved ones, cannot dress himself, cannot bathe himself, cannot wipe himself, and cannot prepare his own food. It is not my God's intention that I would live my last days like this. My God intends for me to live my last days sharing my service, wisdom, knowledge, understanding, life's experiences with my children, my grandchildren, and my great grandchildren.

That I may never be a burden to them in my last days and that I would be a blessing to them. This is why fasting is important. Fasting not only regularly gives your organs and digestive system a rest, but it also plays an active role in reversing these negative effects of aging.

"When you have been stricken by illness, your new car, your new home, your new bank account balance, your work, all of these fade into unimportance until you have regained your vigor and zest for living again."

Remember the last time you were sick and how you felt? You were into yourself, not able to interact with and be a blessing to others, because you were in such discomfort. That is not how we should spend our last days. I am especially concerned with my brain and ability to have good mental clarity and mental retention. I don't want to grow old not recognizing my family members because I have dementia or Alzheimer's disease. It has been estimated that 50 percent of seniors over the age of seventy will have some symptoms of Alzheimer's "in a short time to come."

A study by the *British Journal of Psychiatry* reports that people who ate a plant-based diet reduced their chances of suffering from depression. Conversely, they said a diet of processed meats, sweetened desserts, fried foods, refined cereals, and high-fat dairy products seems to be deleterious for depression. Diabetics have an increased risk of mental decline, dementia, and Alzheimer's, due to the excess sweets and animal products they eat. This can also lead to strokes. According to the most recent studies, filtered coffee (just two cups a day) may be helpful to the body. Coffee may protect against Parkinson's, Alzheimer's, and diabetes, according to recent studies. A group of women were analyzed, and it was determined that after the age of seventy, those who drank coffee most of their lives had better memory retention and memory clarity than those who drank no coffee.

Excess stress in your life can cause brain damage; it destroys brain cells and impairs the growth of new brain cells. This is shown by impaired memory. If you wake up in the middle of the night thinking and worrying about people and problems, it will cause insomnia, and that leads to brain damage. The brain, for proper function, needs the proper rest. The Bible says, "Cast your cares upon me for I careth for you." Don't allow those painful thoughts to keep you from getting proper sleep. It seems that the older you get, the more this problem exists. You must take authority over your thoughts and not entertain the stinking-thinking!

Dr. Caroline Leaf states in her book *Switch On Your Brain*: "Research shows that the vast majority of mental and physical illness comes from our thought-life rather than the environment and genes. Other studies dealing with obsessive compulsive disorders and schizophrenia show definite changes in the brain from the negative to the positive when thinking is brought under control. Some scientists even describe these neuropsychiatric manifestations almost as though negative, toxic thinking opens a gate that allows negative emotions to overwhelm them. And because mind changes matter, this negative thinking changes the brain structure."

The flesh is dumb; it doesn't have a mind of its own. But we listen to our flesh and submit to the weaknesses. So our palate runs our life and controls us. It is time to tell the body: *You will submit. I am the boss.* Remember, what you *think* determines what you *do*.

There have been some nights, when I have awoken in the middle of the night with negative thoughts dancing around in my mind. For example, thoughts of someone who offended me, a disappointment that occurred, a disobedient child, etc., I immediately begin thinking and naming everything to be thankful for, and the list is endless. For example, thank you, God, for the wonderful warm bed; thank you for the fleece blanket; thank you for my family (and name them); thank you for my work and the ability to pay my bills; thank you for my brain; thank you that I wake up pain-free; thank you for my health. These are a few examples. With that, I promise you the ugly thoughts go away, because remember, you can't think two thoughts at the same time. Stress is probably one of the greatest detriments to optimum health. This is determined by what you think. Don't let your thoughts bring on the tension to your body. The choice is yours.

Dr. Caroline Leaf also wrote the following:

> *God designed humans to observe our own thoughts of those that are bad and get rid of them. The importance of capturing those thoughts cannot be underestimated. When you objectively observe your own thinking with the view to capturing rogue thoughts, you*

*in effect direct your attention to stop
the negative impact and rewire healthy
new circuits into your brain.*

It is important to keep in mind that the power of your thoughts will establish either joy or misery. Because of my faith, I personally take authority over a negative thought that keeps returning with of statement: "I take authority over this thought and rebuke it in the name of Jesus." I promise it will go away, but sometimes it can return. If it does return, I will then repeat the statement.

Brain scans will show the difference of one that is negative and one that is positive. It is amazing to see the difference between a healthy brain and an unhealthy brain. One picture really is worth a thousand words. Brain scans and double-blind studies have shown that negative thoughts break down the brain. When we think thoughts that are kind, loving, or positive, we are creating neurons and making the brain healthy. We can decide to do something that is beneficial to our body and brain by eating God-made natural foods, fasting, and detox, and we can overcome the lethargy and weakness of not wanting to fast. We can have victory over our bodies with our thoughts, and we can make the decision to fast and overcome the weakness of our bodies' desires. Like the T-shirt says: *just do it.*

J. Robert Hatherill, PhD, wrote the book *The Brain Gate*. It is such a great book; I could not put it down. I learned so much. He talks about the blood-brain barrier. He states that the brain has the ability to prevent toxins and impurities from entering in. When we eat foods that are fried, animal products, processed foods, dairy, and certain oils that contain bad fats and trans fats, this will do damage to the brain. Bad oils transport toxins such as aluminum, mercury, lead, etc. to the brain. Oils such as corn oil, vegetable oil, canola oil, and sunflower oil are bad oils. Good oils are sesame seed oil, coconut oil, flaxseed oil, cold press olive oil, hemp oil, soy bean oil, and walnut oil.

Risk factors for Alzheimer's disease according to *The Brain Gate* are as follows: brain injury (trauma), pesticide exposure, heavy metal exposure (cadmium, lead, mercury, aluminum), heart disease, high blood pressure, age, gender (females have increased incidence), and animal products. Remember, it is *what* we are putting into our bodies, not how much. "Researchers have shown that aluminum can cross the brain gate barrier and cause nerve cell death. Silica-rich foods such as carrots block the intake of aluminum from the gut." Fish is one of the worst foods to eat for the brain because it has large amounts of mercury and PCBs. I read in the *San Diego Union Tribune* recently that there is a large layer of DDT at the bottom of the San Diego bay. DDT is a pesticide that was banned in United States back in the early 1980s.

There have been forty new diseases since 1970. There is a new disease being discovered every year. Right now, we have 5.5 million people with Alzheimer's disease and two hundred thousand under age sixty-five. It is estimated that there will be twenty million more Alzheimer cases in the next twenty years and that 50 percent of folks over seventy years old will have some symptoms of Alzheimer's by midcentury. Every thirty-three seconds, a new case of Alzheimer's is expected to develop. This costs the United States $259 billion, and the global cost of Alzheimer's and dementia combined reaches $605 billion; by 2020, costs are estimated to reach $1.1 trillion for dementia alone. Symptoms include loss of recognition of their loved ones, repetitive conversation, and the absence of the ability to carry an intelligent conversation. The condition gets progressively worse. I cry when I think of my precious stepmother who had dementia. She was one of the most wonderful human beings I have known, and this dreaded disease simply took her from this world.

Do you want to live your last days like this? I don't! I believe my God wants me to live my senior days being a blessing to others and to pass on my wisdom and love to my loved ones and my fellow man. I want to be able to give my great grandchildren piggy back rides and teach them words of wisdom in all areas of life. This is how I am supposed to live my last days. We all can live like this, but it depends on what we are putting into our bodies and minds. Remember, our bodies are not garbage dumps (garbage in, garbage out), our bodies are God's temple. Yes, you are what you eat. Toxic foods and prescription drugs cause brain shrinkage. Eat God-made natural foods, organic, and you shall have a more abundant life!

CHAPTER 10

Spiritual Fasting

Fasting and prayer is the only proper reason for abstinence from the marital relationship. No exercise, TV, parties, etc.

—1 Corinthians 7:5

Fasting Results

- Initiates a release of spiritual power by removing spiritual hindrances
- Establishes that our God is not our belly
- Creates clarity of mind
- Brings closeness to God

- Gives us victory over fleshly desires and diminishes the power of the flesh over us
- Helps us overcome unbelief and doubt and shows us what we are capable of
- Builds our spiritual life and increases the ability of our mind to react with God's spirit and gives us a new anointing and a closer walk with Jesus
- Makes us more sensitive to the leading of God's Holy Spirit. This enables us to operate more in the realm of his Holy Spirit
- Helps us to receive the outpouring of his spirit that Christ has declared we would have
- Brings answers to prayer, God's best for us, divine guidance
- Brings clarity of mind
- Creates closeness to God
- Helps us break habits
- Humbles us
- Brings deliverance from strongholds
- Brings salvation for others and loved ones
- Can bring miracles
- Sets captives free and loose the bonds of wickedness
- Brings protection

- Encourages repentance
- Encourages mercy
- Brings healing and health
- Ministry involvements or considerations
- Changes the mind of God from destruction to rescue
- Keeps us submissive
- Receives revelation from God
- Encourages and strengthens our faith
- Undoes heavy burdens
- Brings courage and wisdom
- Aids mourning
- Changes our attitude and character to be more Christlike
- God will talk to us, and we will hear from him like never before

What Is Spiritual Fasting from a Biblical Perspective?

Fasting is taught and practiced in both the Old and the New Testaments. Moses, Joshua, Samuel, and all of Israel fasted at one time or another. Fasting is mentioned seventy-four times in the Bible. Elijah, Ezra, Nehemiah, Esther, Daniel, and Apostle Paul all fasted and received a powerful God-blessed strategy for their leadership and their decisions. This is still needed today in the church and the synagogue. Fasting for spiritual purposes is abstinence from food, only drinking water or juices. You will then be fed with spiritual food, the power of the Holy Spirit. The fleshly needs are put into submission, allowing the spiritual to surface, drawing us closer to the God of the universe.

God is calling people to fast. Fasting regularly increases our ability to hear from God walk in his ways and do his will, ultimately having control over the flesh. When fasting, some folks have testified that they receive a divine guidance and a loving closeness to our Lord like they have never had before. We experience the concentrated, intensified power of God that can work in our lives through fasting. Famous people like Charles Finney and Charles Spurgeon, who practiced fasting regularly, became great soul-winning preachers and world changers. People can achieve mighty levels of wisdom, knowledge, and understanding through fasting and prayer.

Fasting humbles our soul and masters our flesh, our appetite, and manifests intense desire to seek

God. It gives us power over demonic evil spiritual oppression and aids in our prayer life. Isaiah 58:6–12 states:

Is not this the fast that I have chosen to loose the bonds of wickedness, to undo the heavy burdens, and to let the oppressed go free, and that you break every yoke. Is it not to share your bread with the hungry, and that you bring the poor that are cast out back to your home, when you see the naked you clothe him. Then shall your light break forth as the morning and shine, and your health will spring forth speedily: and your righteousness shall go before you: the glory of the Lord shall be your reward. Then you shall call and the Lord will answer. You shall cry and he will say: Here I am. If you take away from the midst of you the yoke, the putting forth of the finger, and speaking vanity, and if you satisfy the afflicted soul then shall your light rise in obscurity and your darkness be as the noon day. And the Lord will guide you continually and satisfy your soul in drought and make you healthy. You will be like a watered garden and like a spring of water. You will be the restorer of paths to dwell in.

Fasting is a biblical practice that has three amazing benefits that happens to us in body mind and spirit. If you need to make a decision in your life, possibly marriage or a job, fasting is in order.

I was engaged to a man for seven years. He wanted to get married, but I felt something was just holding me back. I went to a place called Prayer Mountain, owned by the Koreans. I stayed in a little bungalow for seven days and locked myself away. I fasted on water and prayed and sought the Lord about whether I should marry this man or not. The third day into my fast, I heard an audible voice deep in my heart. He said to me: "Millan, the problem is not him, the problem is you." You see, I thought that he had so many problems that were the reasons I could not marry him. I knew that was God speaking to me because I didn't think *I* had any problems. God does not hold back anything but truth. I was a problem, and he told me so during my fast. I did not want to hear this. But I knew it was from the Lord. At the end of that seven-day fast, I knew that I was not to marry this man. I found out later that he was unfaithful and would have been a complete adulterer during our marriage. This is something that I had not been aware of.

There was a case of a pastor who had cancer, and his church fasted and prayed, and within a week, the cancer was gone. In the 1960s, there was a great drought in America. Crops and livestock were dying, and farmers were suffering horribly. President Johnson called the nation to a time of fasting and prayer, and in three days, the heavens broke open, and the rain came down and America was spared.

I believe that most of us who believe have a problem with faith, but God's word says that faith will produce knowledge, self-control, moral excellence, godliness, perseverance, brotherly kindness, and love. Fasting is a very important part of accomplishing this kind of faith. Fasting does for us mentally what it does for us physically; it removes toxic thoughts from our minds. It humbles our soul and gives us a fresh sensitivity to the God of the universe. Fasting will allow us to deny what we want and embrace what God wants. His ways are so very perfect. True fasting brings humility that cares only about what God thinks and wants for us. By fasting, we put our spirit in charge of our minds.

Fasting somehow improves our ability to handle frustration and the stresses of life. God confirms that in his Word. Do you get frustrated, as I do, about what we see going on today in our culture? Doesn't it make sense that if we prayed and fasted for our nation that would move the hand of God? It truly is hard to hear from God when our flesh is stuffed with food and we are feeling lethargic and want to take a nap. Think about it: we are constantly being ruled by our flesh. What we see, what we taste, what we hear, what we do, what we feel, pleasures of the flesh, etc. Putting that into submission and taking control over it open up heaven's gate to allow a spiritual realm to take effect, to allow the hand of God to move, and to experience more of the spiritual realm and hear the voice of God.

When Should One Fast?

Whenever God speaks to you. Whenever you have a concern. Whenever you have an emotionally stressful time. Whenever you are attacked verbally. Or otherwise, whenever you need to make a decision that is very important. Whenever you care for someone's soul. When you fast, expect a spiritual reward. When you fast and pray, expect answers. Sometimes, God will speak to you audibly. You will receive guidance before, during, and after your fast. Remember that when you fast on a regular basis, you always have control over your flesh and your appetite. Your needs will always be supplied and met. Did you know that relationships that have gone foul or sour can always be restored through fasting and prayer? You will come into overflowing abundance.

Results in Fasting

Here are some wonderful rewards. You can obey the Lord God with greatest of ease; you can obtain divine revelation. You will have incredible health. You will have a shared experience in the glory of

God. Difficult times and heavy burdens will be eliminated. Any addictions or bad habits can be broken; your prayers will be answered quickly. You will have the guidance of Almighty God on a continual basis. Feeling hopeless and desolate will be changed to feeling victorious.

Fasting humbles our spirit, and God desires us to be humble. Fasting helps us to consider others more important than ourselves. Fasting gives us the ability to consider others and their needs more than our own. Fasting enables us to get the wisdom of God's knowledge and also his understanding, placing you in the spiritual glory. Fasting will help us to truly understand the real meaning of love for our fellow man and love for God. Remember that fasting will expand God's power, and we will sense it in our lives and be more aware of his presence.

Miracles Resulting from Those Who Have Fasted

Mahesh Chavda, the author of *Prayer and Fasting*, shared his experience in the miracle of a boy by the name of Stevie, who had Down syndrome and severe mental illness.

He was sixteen years old and he was a self-mutilator who was driven to cry out and beat himself in his face constantly. The psychologist advocated administering electric shock therapy to Stevie for six months. This was meant to modify Stevie's behavior and prevent him from beating himself. His face felt like dry alligator skin because he beat himself continually. Many times, they would find him with blood streaming from his nose lips and mouth.

Since I worked at this institution, I would come to him and Stevie could sense God's love coming from me and he would put his head on my shoulder and just weep. Finally, I said: Lord, you told me that you would send me here to love these children. What is the answer for Stevie? The Holy Spirit said: *this kind goes not out but by prayer and fasting. Now pray and fast for Stevie.*

I fasted for fourteen days on water. I went to the institution where

Stevie lived after that I took Stevie into my little office cubicle and said: "Stevie I know your mind may not understand what I'm saying, but your spirit is eternal. I want to tell you that I am a servant of the Lord Jesus Christ. I have come to preach good news to you. I want you to know that Jesus Christ came to set the captives free." Remember, Stevie is severely mentally ill. Then I said: "in the name of Jesus, you evil spirit of mutilation, you let him go now."

Suddenly Stevie's body was flung about eight feet away from me and hit the other wall of the cubicle. When Stevie hit the wall, his body was elevated about three feet above the floor. Then he slid down to the floor and let out a long sigh. Immediately I smelled an incredibly foul smell of rotten eggs and burning sulfur in the room which gradually faded away. I quickly went to Stevie, cradled him in my arms and removed his splints the doctors had put on his arms to keep him from hitting himself. He watched with wide eyes. Then Stevie began to bend his arms and gently feel his face. I watched him softly touch his eyes his nose and his ears then he started sobbing. I realize that for the first time he was not being driven to beat himself. He was gently touching his face and he had been delivered. In that unforgettable moment, the Lord revealed to me what a powerful weapon he had given us to pull down strongholds and set the captives free through fasting and prayer. Within a few months, all the scabs had fallen off Stevie's face he had begun to heal because he had stopped beating himself.

You can change the condition and the destiny of your city, and even your nation, by joining God's end time army of men and women committed to fasting and prayer. Countries that have been under the domain of communism have fasted in unison for the release of communistic stronghold in their country and were granted freedom from communism. Demonic spirits get very uncomfortable when believers begin fasting. I believe there is no sickness that cannot be recovered through fasting. Demonic spirits cannot stay around when a person is fasting because there is a totally different atmosphere that is open to the freedom of God's Holy Spirit. These spirits tremble when a person fasts and prays.

In *Only Love Can Make a Miracle*, Chavda wrote the following regarding an acquaintance and her husband. He had gone to their house with his friend, whom he wanted to bring to salvation. This friend was having many problems and wanted nothing to do with Jesus.

> *As we pulled into the driveway, a woman—I could only assume it was our hostess—suddenly ran out the front door screaming, 'He's killing my husband! He's killing my husband!'*
>
> She was hysterical. Skip and I raced into the house. We didn't see anyone there. For a moment, we couldn't figure out what was going

on. All the while, the woman kept screaming, "You've got to stop him! He's killing my husband!" We ran to the kitchen in the back of the house.

Then we saw it.

In the backyard was a man. Again, I assumed it must be the husband. He was leaning against a tree, barely able to stay upright. His clothes were shredded and spattered with blood. One of his arms was slashed open from shoulder to elbow so badly that you could see the exposed bone. He was a frightful sight.

Even more frightful was the dog a few feet in front of him. A big dog. Probably the biggest German Shepherd I have ever seen, certainly the biggest I ever want to see. It was growling and snarling menacingly, crouched down as if on the verge of attacking again.

I tried to figure out what to do. I was in no hurry to mess with that dog. But the wife was continuing to cry and scream frantically, and it was clear the man wasn't going to survive another attack by that vicious dog.

In a split second, I made up my mind. I had to do something to help this man, to try to save his life. I rushed to the side door of the house. As I did, I noticed a broom leaning up against the wall. I grabbed it and headed for the back yard.

Just inside the fence was a patio with some folding lawn furniture arranged on it. I picked up one of the chairs. I must have been thinking of the lion-tamers I had seen in circuses. Maybe I could keep the dog at bay long enough for the man to escape. Slowly, I edged toward the dog, holding the broom and the chair out in front of me.

Suddenly, I heard the Holy Spirit speak to me: "*Bind it.*"

"Bind it?" What did that mean? How did I go about "binding" something? What should I bind?

The words came again. "*Bind it!*"

The dog had now turned its attention toward me. I looked down at those crazed eyes, those ferocious teeth. Without really understanding what I was saying or why, I just stared back at the dog and said in a sharp, tense voice, "I bind you in the name of Jesus!"

Suddenly, a tremendous peace and calm came over me. All the fear just drained away. Something inside me seemed to sense that the danger was past now, that everything was under control.

The man was still slumped against the tree, just barely able to keep from falling over. I moved slowly, cautiously in his direction, all the time watching the dog. The dog seemed different somehow. He was still snarling, still growling, still crouched as if to spring. But he seemed unable to move, as if his muscles had frozen. As if he wanted

to jump but couldn't. As if he were…
bound.

Finally, I made it to the tree. I reached out to steady the man, and he simply fainted and collapsed in my arms. Apparently, the fear and loss of blood were just too much for him. I tossed the broomstick over the fence, bent down, and hoisted him over my shoulder. I couldn't get back to the house without going past the dog, so I decided to just head for the fence. I used the chair to help me climb over into the neighbor's yard and lay the man down on the grass.

He was out cold and looked terribly pale. He had lost a great deal of blood, and the horrible gash in his arm was still bleeding. Someone brought me a towel, and with the towel and the broomstick, I made a tourniquet for his arm, to try to stop the bleeding.

I heard an ambulance pulling up in front. Apparently Skip or the wife or one of the neighbors had thought to call for it. Thanks be to God!

My moment of rejoicing was obliterated by a sudden flash of panic. I realized the man wasn't breathing! I put my hand on his chest, hoping to detect some slight rising and falling movement. Nothing. I grabbed his wrist and felt for a pulse. Nothing there either.

"O please, God," I prayed inwardly. "You can't let this happen. You can't just let him die." I was beginning to get a sneaking suspicion as to why the Lord had told me to come to Dallas. "I can't believe you brought me here just to see this man die."

The paramedics were coming through the gate now. I felt his chest again. Still nothing! I prayed earnestly, "O God, please."

Just then he let out a sigh. I was so happy, I almost fainted. As the paramedics lifted him onto the stretcher, he regained consciousness just for a moment. He opened his eyes and looked toward me.

"Can this man come with us?" He asked the paramedics. "He just saved my life." Then he blacked out again.

Skip and I rode with him to the hospital. We paced around and around the waiting room until a doctor finally came and told us his friend would be alright. We collapsed into our chairs like a couple of limp dishrags.

We sat there for a moment in silence, then Skip turned and looked at me. "That was amazing," he said. "Really amazing. I was so scared I couldn't do a thing, but you just walked out there as if you weren't afraid of anything; as if you weren't even afraid of dying. I've never met anyone with so much peace. What's your secret?"

At that moment, at long last, the Lord said to me, "*Now.*"

I shared with Skip about the God who loved me, who loved him, who loved all of us so much that he sent his Son, Jesus, to die for us so that we could live forever. I told him that God wanted us to enjoy fellowship with Him forever, but that our sins stood in the way. I told him that anyone who wanted could turn from their sin, welcome Jesus into their life as their Savior and Lord, and receive the gift of new life in His Holy Spirit. I told him that the moment they did this, they received not only the promise of eternal salvation, but also the promise of joy and of a peace that surpasses understanding even in this life.

I told Skip that if this was what he wanted, he could pray with me right then and there to receive Jesus into his heart. It was and he did.

God's word says we fast to humble ourselves before God and obtain his grace and power. Fasting purifies us and enables us to be honest, have power, be humble, make proper decisions, receive God's grace, overcome, and be obedient; let go and let God.

I find that there have been times when I felt in my life complete inability to conquer a habit I had and could not stop. I think of my diabetes and my sugar cravings that I had many years ago. Now I know that fasting and prayer have given me victory over these habitual weaknesses that are a detriment to me physically, mentally, and spiritually. I think this is a great miracle in my own life.

I would encourage each one of you who may feel desolate and hopeless in whatever circumstance you are in to consider a fasting and prayer regimen. Perhaps you know someone in your family or friends who is addicted to drugs or pornography and has mental issues like depression, anger, or rebelliousness. The list goes on and on. I promise that if you fast and pray, the hand of God will move to deliver, rescue, heal, restore, and give hope once more. Remember, God is teaching us to love each other, to love God with all our mind, our heart, and our soul. This is what Jesus taught: *love*. Love is truly serving each other and truly caring about others. Fasting clears our heart, mind, and soul. The process helps us accomplish attributes, such as love and healing. In order to be physically and emotionally healthier, we should all make fasting a regular part of our lives.

CHAPTER 11

Testimonial

Israel fasted in repentance. Israelites felt God left them for twenty years. Samuel said "get rid of your god images." Then God rescued them from Philistine attack.
—1 Samuel 7:3

Could our god be junk food, the food that causes sickness and disease?

Dear Millan,

As a person who is over sixty years old and [has] been concerned with the quality of my health as I grow older, I would like to say how much I appreciated your fasting retreat. As you know, my primary health concerns were detox of the body and removal of parasites. I was very pleased to see round worms from small to large, twenty-four to thirty inches, make their way out. Obviously, your experience and skill contributed greatly to the results. Your detox program along with some herbs for parasites certainly [have] helped me regain my body's health and well-being. Additionally, I would like to thank you for seeing to our personal needs such as lodging, internet access, transportation to and from the airport, and the overnight stay in Julian Mountains. Taking time to see to our comforts meant a lot to us. Until we see each other again, take care and live well.

Sincerely,
GG from Washington State

Fasting is outstanding when one is trying to be healthy as you have read in the previous chapters. I want to refer here to a gentleman by the name of Roy White. When he was 106 years old, he looked like he was sixty; his secret was fasting four times a year for seven days each time and doing progressive weight training three times a week.

At the age of seventy, Martin Nick was playing a champion tennis game with much younger players, and he was winning. What was his secret? Regular fasting. He said he feels like a twenty-year-old there on the court. The number of health benefits fasting brings is great at any age; actress Cloris Leachman states that fasting is simply wonderful. It is a miracle cure. Benjamin Franklin advised to lessen your meals and lengthen your life.

In his book, *Miracle of Fasting*, Paul Bragg shares his story of hiring ten husky athletes to hike in Death Valley in very high temperatures for the whole day. Paul Bragg had been fasting for thirty days on just water, and on this day, they brought a station wagon full of sandwiches, salt tablets, sodas, etc. for the other hikers to eat. Halfway through the hike, half of them collapsed and could not continue the hike. By the end of the day's journey, they all failed to continue the hike, some even vomiting and having to be taken away in an ambulance. Paul Bragg slept in the desert that night by himself, got up the next morning, and hiked all the way back by himself, drinking only distilled water. He was a grandfather at the time.

Sylvia Franco was a medical doctor and had a master's degree in business by the time she was thirty years old. She kept in shape and ate properly, but she and her husband couldn't seem to conceive a child. She spent $100,000 on fertility treatments but to no avail. Finally, she contacted a doctor who found that Sylvia was in a toxic condition and that was messing up her hormones. The doctor concluded that taking birth control pills for five years and several doses of an unusual type of antibiotic had upset her system. When she quit taking the birth control pills, her hormone levels became unbalanced. He put her on a cleansing fast, and in three months, she conceived a child. Thomas Edison states the doctor of the future will give no medicine but will instruct his patients in the care of the human frame, in diet, and in the cause and prevention of disease.

There are so many people in our culture today who suffer from depression and are taking medications for that reason. At my fasting retreat, every other person that comes has suffered or is suffering from depression. If one would only fast and cleanse, the depression concerns would be eradicated. Fasting clears the mind and can release us from mental disorders. In a Moscow psychiatric unit, seven thousand patients had disorders ranging from schizophrenia to neurosis. They were treated with conventional medicine, but nothing seemed to help. The directors decided that they would try what they called a "hunger experiment." They did not feed these patients solid food for a week giving them only water and juice. After that week, more than 80 percent of those patients were well enough to be released and lived normal lives. In Japan, a medical journal reported that out of 382 patients with psychiatric diseases, 87 percent were cured through the use of fasting.

Dr. Gabriel Cousins MD says: "I have often observed in the fasting participants that by four days of fasting, concentration seems to improve, creativity expands, depression lifts, insomnia stops, anxieties fade, the mind becomes more tranquil and a natural joy begins to appear."

"It is my hypothesis that when the physical toxins are cleared from the brain cells, brain function automatically and significantly improves and spiritual capacities expands. Sleeping while on a fast is very rejuvenating." Dr. Cott states, "A good reason to fast is to lose weight, [it is] the quickest way to save money, to lower blood pressure and cholesterol levels, to sleep better, to digest food better, to save time, to regulate bowels, to learn better eating habits and to call attention on social issues. There are of course many more benefits. Fasting is the most effective way to kill unwanted parasites, bacteria, viruses, and fungi."

Trisha Bragg states, "Fasting is not starving. It's nature's cure that God has given us." She fasts every Monday and the first three days of each month. It's a precious time for body, mind, and soul and for cleansing and renewal. The elimination of waste from fasting will increase your longevity.

Dr. Elson Haas MD says that "Fasting is the single greatest healing therapy. When I first discovered fasting many years ago, I felt as if it had saved my life and transformed my illness into health. I believe fasting is the missing link in the Western diet."

In Dr. Cott's book, he discusses a very obese man who wanted to feel human again and fasted for fourteen consecutive weekends. Then he fasted for one day a week for nine months. Over the years' time, he cut his weight exactly in half, going from 360 pounds to 180 pounds.

Cott talks about a post-hospitalization questionnaire that was sent to over 709 obese individuals who had fasted at the University of Pennsylvania hospital, whose pioneer fasting program was supervised by Dr. Garfield Duncan. Of the 50 percent who responded, approximately 46 percent had continued to lose weight, and 21 percent had regained at the reduced level at which they had completed their fast.

A client of mine had melanoma cancer that had metastasized. The doctors sent her home to die. She stayed at our retreat for two weeks, went back to the MDs to be tested, and her cancer was in remission. Another had breast cancer, stayed one week, went back home, was tested, and cancer was in remission.

According to Dr. Paavo Airola, there was a woman who was fifty-four years old, had painful arthritis, and was grossly overweight. She was put on a liquid fast for 249 days and lost 74 of her 262 pounds. As a pleasant side effect, her arthritis went away. He also tells of another woman who fasted and lost fifty-two pounds on a forty-four-day fast; she actually went from size twenty to a size twelve. I had a lady stay at my fasting retreat who was grossly overweight, weighed 250 pounds and lost 50 pounds in seven days doing the juice fast, cleansing herbal program, and colon cleansing.

"After a fast, your mind becomes so powerful that it can take full control of the body. It becomes the complete master, and if a person does not go back to his old habits, he can maintain this mastery of the body for the rest of his life. Fasting instills personal confidence. Fasting gives a person a positive mental attitude. Fasting promotes tranquility of mind and a glow of wellbeing that no other therapy can offer. Fasting renovates, revives, and purifies every one of the trillions of cells that make up the body. Fasting is the royal road to internal purity," says Paul Bragg, as written in his book, *Miracle of Fasting*.

After a seven-day fast, you will start to notice how your body feels lighter; your mind becomes very sharp, your memory improves with great clarity, and you will desire to walk or exercise. This is a result of your insides becoming more cleansed and your body becoming healthier and more youthful.

I want to tell you about a previous love of my life. He was an ultramarathon runner. He ran the one hundred-mile races. I put him on a two-week fast, cleansing herbs, and colon hydrotherapy. Yes, he lost a few pounds, but after the two-week period, he bulked up with healthy eating for another one hundred-mile race, and then he ran the race and came in second. He was rated the seventeenth top runner of the United States. That was phenomenal for him, as he had never made that kind of accomplishment before fasting. So if you need to make some decisions, or plans for accomplishments in your life that are important to you like a new job or a marriage, something that requires a lot from you, I suggest you fast prior for clarity, for wisdom, for knowledge, and for understanding.

I suggest, before you start your journey of fasting, to stand naked in front of a mirror and take a good hard look. What do you see? Is your skin saggy? Do you have cellulite, wrinkles? How about your muscles? Are there any? Are you overweight? Do you like what you see? How about how you feel? Do you wake up in the morning dreading getting out of bed? Are you hungry all the time? Are you tired all the time? Are you angry, bitter, or unsatisfied in any way? Do you sleep well at night? Do you wake up in the middle of the night thinking negative thoughts? Are you urinating all night long? How about your bowels? Are you constipated? Do you have diarrhea? Do you have an itching anus? Do you look forward to the new day with dread? These are questions that need good answers. And I can tell you that the answer is fasting. Yes, it will require discipline and, maybe in your eyes, deprivation. But it will give you discipline and a new lease on life as you have never known before.

Seven-day Fasting Results

Name	Waist (inches lost)	Hips (inches lost)	Total weight lost
Patricia	3	1	8 1/4
Gina	4 1/4	1 1/4	9 1/4
Steve	2 1/4	1 1/2	11 1/2
Aletheia	2	3/4	4 3/4
Joann	4	1	8
Erin	3	1	5 1/4

Name	Waist (inches lost)	Hips (inches lost)	Total weight lost
Christiana	2 1/4	2 1/4	8 3/4
Tim	2	0	9 3/4
Sandra	1	1	5 3/4
Heather	4 1/4	1 3/4	14 3/4
Judy	3	1 1/2	11
Mary	3	3/4	7 1/2
Tonia	2	1/4	7 1/4
Nabil	2	2 1/2	8 1/2
Sherine	2 1/4	1	8 1/2
John	2 1/4	1	7
Donna	4	2	14 1/4
Tracy	3	3/4	11
Lena	1 1/4	0	3
Lisa	2	1	7
Caroline	2 3/4	1 3/4	7 1/2
Donna	3	1 1/2	7 1/2
Darci	3	1/2	6 1/4
Judy	1	1 1/2	10 3/4
Susan	1 3/4	1 3/4	10 1/4
Shelly	3 1/2	3 1/4	8 1/2
Barbara	2 1/2	2	6 1/4
Karen	3 1.4	2	10

Name	Waist (inches lost)	Hips (inches lost)	Total weight lost
Diane	3 3/4	2 1/2	8 3/4
Patrica	1 1/2	2	5
Diane	1	1/4	5 1/2
Marlene	2	1 1/2	8
Sue	1	1 1/4	10 1/2
Douglas	3 3/4	1 1/4	7
Autumn	4 1/2	1 1/2	10
Francesca	8 1/2	1 1/2	5
Heidi	2	3/4	5
Sarah	1	1/2	2 1/2
Susan	2 3/4	4	8
Marina	3/4	0	6
Barbara	2 1/2	1	11
Pris	2	1 1/4	3
Fiona	13	17	7 3/4
Kalina	3/4	1	5
Emily	4 1/2	1/4	3 3/4
Donna	2 3/4	1	6
Conda	2 3/4	1/2	5 1/2
Donna	2 1/4	1 3/4	13 3/4
Jennifer	1/2	3/4	1/2
Diane	1 1/2	1	4 1/4

Name	Waist (inches lost)	Hips (inches lost)	Total weight lost
Sean	3/4	2 1/4	11
Diane	1 1/4	1	7
Sylvia	3	3/4	17
Sharon	2	1 1/4	8 1/2
Maggie	3 3/4	2 1/2	7
Monalina	2 1/4	1	6 1/2
Della	2 1/2	1/2	7
Margaret	5	1	9
Victoria	3	1/2	5
Bo	3/4	1 3/4	5 3/4
Betty	3/4	1 1/4	7
Claude	2	3/4	10
Saul	3	1 1/4	10
Jaclyn	1 1/2	1	4 1/2
Lou	2 1/2	1	9 1/4
Francesca	2 1/2	1/2	6
Marcus	3 1/4	1 1/2	5
Linda	1	3/4	6
John	2	1 1/2	10 1/4
Stephen	2 3/4	0	10
Judy	1 1/4	1 1/4	6
Galina	2 3/4	1 1/4	9

Name	Waist (inches lost)	Hips (inches lost)	Total weight lost
Inessa	1 1/2	0	10
Laurel	3/4	1 1/2	8
Karla	1 1/4	0	5 1/4
Juana	1 1/2	3/4	6
Alexandra	1 3/4	1 3/4	9
Jilly	3	1 1/4	7
Lou	2	3/4	6
Debra	1	3/4	5
Jane	4 1/4	1/4	4
Lean	1	2	7 1/2
Leeah	1	3/4	6
Marie	2 3/4	0	5
Dean	1 1/4	2 1/4	8 1/2
Margaret	1 1/4	3/4	12
Robert	3/4	3/4	7
Walter	2	3/4	13
Linda	2 1/2	1	3
Lano	1 3/4	1 1/4	7 1/4
Frank	1 1/2	1 1/4	8
Beth	3/4	1 1/2	4 3/4
David	1	1 1/4	11
Cory	2	0	7

Name	Waist (inches lost)	Hips (inches lost)	Total weight lost
Jon	3 1/2	2	7 1/2
Cathy	3/4	1 1/2	3 1/2
Jennifer	1 1/2	1/2	5
Erika	2 1/2	1	3 1/4
Sheila	2 1/2	1/2	9
Gary	1 3/4	1 1/2	8
Marsha	1/4	1/4	2 1/2
Jaclyn	1 1/4	1 1/2	1 1/2
Cheryl	1/2	1 1/4	7
Shana	3/4	1/2	1
Diane	1/2	1 1/2	5
Suzi	3 1/4	1/2	3
Marlene	2	1	10
Jenn	2 3/4	1/2	9
Angie	2	1 1/4	3
Mary	2 1/2	6	12
Hank	1 1/2	3/4	9 1/2
Dawn	1	3/4	4
Chelsea	2	1	6
Catherine	2 3/4	3/4	9 1/2
Eric	4 3/4	1	21 1/2
Anne	1 1/2	1 1/4	8

Name	Waist (inches lost)	Hips (inches lost)	Total weight lost
Rachel	1 3/4	1/2	7
Gail	0	1/2	8
Donn	4 3/4	3/4	11 1/2
Mary	1 3/4	1 3/4	11
Jaqueline	4 1/2	3/4	11
Noemie	4	2	0

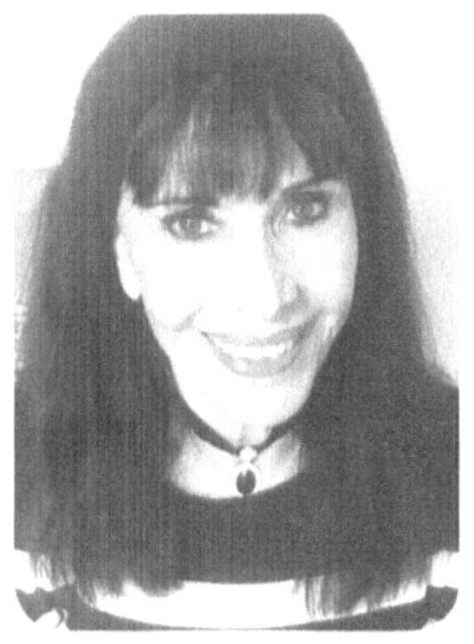

Millan Chessman, BS, CCT, began her pioneering journey in the alternative health field in 1970. What began as a personal pursuit to resolve her health challenges evolved into a successful practice guiding over thirty thousand clients, many with dramatic health improvement, through fasting, nutrition, internal cleansing, and detoxification.

This senior dynamic and possibly the only licensed great grandmother Zumba instructor authored the first book about modern-day professional Intero Hydrotherapy, *Cleanse Internally*, a national best seller. It has almost one hundred testimonials with before and after photos, showing the power of her successful program. She also published *Vegetarian Delights*, a cookbook of multiethnic recipes for optimal health.

Millan Chessman lives her life (walks the talk) in regular practice of biblical principles, fasting, and following the nutritional guidelines she has espoused for half a century. She is a fasting coach and continues to teach detoxification, weight loss, and nutrition and a program of eating foods designed for the body (God-made foods) at her fasting retreat in El Cajon, California.

Email: millanchessman@gmail.com
Website: www.aonefastingretreat.com
Website: www.millanchessman.com
Telephone: 619-562-5446